PLAY IN HEALTHCARE

The importance of play in children's health and care services, both as a form of therapy and as a distraction, is often overlooked. This unique text promotes developmentally appropriate provision within healthcare settings for children and young people and provides an introduction to the underpinning knowledge and skills.

Covering core content – such as the role of play in child development, relevant anatomy and physiology, the concept of resilience, health promotion, developing appropriate provision and working in diverse healthcare settings – each chapter:

- makes links with the NHS Knowledge and Skills Framework and the Children's Workforce Development Council's Common Core of Skills and Knowledge
- begins with an overview of the chapter objectives
- contains a variety of activities such as reflective exercises, case studies and practical tasks that will promote both skills and knowledge needed in the workplace
- concludes with a selection of additional useful resources and further reading suggestions.

Designed for all healthcare professionals who work with children and young people, including those studying to become healthcare play specialists and children's nurses, this text provides practical examples of how all members of the multidisciplinary team can help to support children's play.

Alison Tonkin is Programme Area Manager for Higher Education in Health and Social Care at S   rd member for the Healthcare
Play Specialist   ollege's foundation degree in
Healthcare Play

This book is clearly aimed at healthcare professionals working with children and young people, to promote the use of therapeutic play and recreation in their working practices. The chapters are written by a number of Hospital Play Specialists, a Community Children's Nurse and those involved in currently training Healthcare Play Specialists. The book is structured in such a way that the reader can read individual chapters or the whole book, depending upon their individual requirements. This flexibility in the design of the book enables readers to gain a greater understanding of any given area of interest related to therapeutic play and its application to the practice setting.

Each chapter is linked to both the NHS Knowledge and Skills Framework, and the Common Core of Skills and Knowledge for the Children's Workforce. Clear objectives are identified for the reader at the start of each chapter. A combination of questions for reflection, and activities related to the themes in each chapter, aid the reader in understanding the main concepts. Theoretical underpinnings are applied to practice, with examples from practice to further illustrate the concepts discussed in the chapter.

All members of the MDT need to work together to give the child and/or young person the best experience when in contact with healthcare professionals. Play is described as the work of the child, and is a tool they use to help make sense of their world. This book gives an excellent overview of the importance of therapeutic play to children and young people, and how it can be incorporated into the routine practices of the MDT in very practical ways. I see this book not only as a key text for Healthcare Play Specialist students, but also as a resource for students and practitioners in other healthcare professions, to aid in understanding the importance of therapeutic play in relation to the health and wellbeing of children and young people. This is a text that I will be recommending to my first and second year pre-registration child health nursing students, and to any healthcare professional interested in giving therapeutic play a greater prominence in their day-to-day practice. It provides not only an understanding of the relevance and uses of therapeutic play, but it also informs the reader of the different areas that make up the role of the healthcare play specialist. This is a vital role, not only in the acute setting, but also in the community setting.

Laila Paulsen-Becejac, MSc, BSc, Associate Degree, RGN, RSCN, RNT, RN
(USA), RNC (NICU – USA),
Senior Lecturer and Academic Link for Collaborative Colleges and Post Reg Offer
(Child Health), College of Nursing, Midwifery and Healthcare,
University of West London, UK

PLAY IN HEALTHCARE

Using play to promote child development and wellbeing

Edited by Alison Tonkin

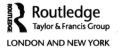

Routledge
Taylor & Francis Group

LONDON AND NEW YORK

First published 2014
by Routledge
2 Park Square, Milton Park, Abingdon, Oxon, OX14 4RN

and by Routledge
711 Third Avenue, New York, NY 10017

Routledge is an imprint of the Taylor & Francis Group, an informa business

British Library Cataloguing in Publication Data
A catalogue record for this book is available from the British Library

Library of Congress Cataloging in Publication Data
Play in healthcare: using play to promote child development and wellbeing/ edited by Alison Tonkin.
 p.; cm.
 Includes bibliographical references.
 I. Tonkin, Alison, 1962 – editor of compilation.
 [DNLM: 1. Play and Playthings–Great Britain. 2. Child–Great Britain.
 3. Child Development–Great Britain. 4. Child Health Services–Great
 Britain. 5. Child, Preschool–Great Britain. WS 105.5.P5]
 RJ102
 362.19892–dc23
 2014000165

ISBN: 978-0-415-71292-7 (hbk)
ISBN: 978-0-415-71293-4 (pbk)
ISBN: 978-1-315-88359-5 (ebk)

Typeset in Bembo
by Wearset Ltd, Boldon, Tyne and Wear

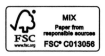
MIX
Paper from
responsible sources
FSC   FSC® C013056
www.fsc.org

Printed and bound in Great Britain by
TJ International Ltd, Padstow, Cornwall

To the memory of Richard Fisher, with love and thanks
'A great teacher and a fine man'

CONTENTS

FIGURES

TABLES

CONTRIBUTORS

Frances Barbour, Health Play Specialist, Lecturer – FdA Healthcare Play Specialism, Stanmore College, Middlesex.

Sandie Dinnen, Vice Principal (Curriculum and Quality), Stanmore College, Middlesex.

Jenni Etchells, Children's Community Nurse, Hertfordshire Community NHS Trust.

Sharon Honey, Director, Health, Care and Social Sciences, Stanmore College, Middlesex.

Norma Jun-Tai, Health Play Specialist, Lecturer in Early Childhood Studies, Nescot College and Kingston University, Surrey.

Vanessa Lovett, Deputy Chief Examiner for Council for Awards in Care, Health and Education (CACHE), Lecturer – FdA Healthcare Play Specialism, Stanmore College, Middlesex.

Irene O'Donnell, Play Services Manager, University College London Hospitals NHS Foundation Trust, Chair, National Association of Health Play Specialists.

Helen Peck, Health Play Specialist, Watford General Hospital, West Hertfordshire Hospitals NHS Trust.

Alison Tonkin, Programme Area Manager for Higher Education in Health and Social Care, Stanmore College, Lecturer – FdA Healthcare Play Specialism, Stanmore College, Middlesex.

Sue Ware, Health Play Specialist, Editor, *The Journal of the National Association of Health Play Specialists*.

Claire Weldon, Lecturer in Health and Social Care, Stanmore College, Middlesex.

Julia Whitaker, Health Play Specialist (Freelance) Registration Coordinator, Healthcare Play Specialist Education Trust.

FOREWORD

This book is a welcome and much needed publication which, for the reader, pulls together all the elements necessary to understand the requirements of children, and young people's needs in respect of their health and wellbeing when experiencing a healthcare setting.

It is a privilege to be invited to contribute a Foreword, particularly as the developing child has been at the heart of my career spanning 22 years in early years education and 18 years in a children's hospital.

It was during my involvement in the training programme for health play specialists that I met the editor of this publication, who shares my belief that well-qualified practitioners will enhance the wellbeing of children and young people in their care.

Since the first funded hospital play worker some 50 years ago, subsequent publications from the Department of Health recommendations and parental pressure there has been a growing awareness by health-related employers of the value of the particular knowledge and skills of an accomplished health play specialist.

Over the decades various groups have campaigned for better access and information for children in hospital, which after the United Nations Convention on the Rights of the Child came into force on 15 January 1992, in the context of this book, embedded a child's and young person's right to health, information, education and play.

With the support of the professional team and families, an experienced practitioner can maintain developmental goals and minimize emotional stress for children and young people when faced with medical admissions and interventions in any healthcare setting.

With the advancement of science, children with some illnesses or conditions have a life expectancy far longer than as little as 25 years ago; however, poor mental health is becoming more prevalent in younger children than ever before. It is therefore vital that children and young people have access to health-related education and play of the highest quality in order to mitigate non-compliance of treatment or deterioration in coping strategies, both of which can lead to a lifetime of misery.

It is fitting that this publication illustrates the breadth of knowledge and understanding of children and young people's needs as they journey towards good health and wellbeing.

Suzanne Storer
Chairman, Healthcare Play Specialist Education Trust

ACKNOWLEDGEMENTS

Alison Tonkin would like to thank:

- All the contributors to this book, including those within Chapter 12, who have given their time so generously in order to share their enthusiasm, knowledge and expertise; we have written this together.
- Suzanne Storer, Chairman of the Healthcare Play Specialist Education Trust, for kindly writing the Foreword for the book and for all her kind support and encouragement since this project began.
- The Senior Management Team at Stanmore College, who enabled this project to be undertaken and completed under their care.
- Friends and colleagues at Stanmore College, who have engaged in this process, offering guidance, suggestions and kind words of encouragement when needed. In particular, Claire Weldon, who continually helps to transform ideas into practical outcomes.
- NHS Employers for allowing descriptions from the KSF core dimensions in Appendix 4 of *Appraisals and KSF made simple: a practical guide* to be reproduced at the beginning of each chapter.
- Louise Kershaw, National College for Teaching and Leadership, for tenaciously tracking down permission to use content from the Children's Workforce Development Council.
- Grace McInnes, Commissioning Editor, Routledge, for giving us the opportunity to write this book after two years of searching for a publisher.
- James Watson, Senior Editorial Assistant, Health and Social Care, Routledge for gently leading and guiding us through this process.
- Debbie Tonkin for proofreading the entire content.
- My family and Irena, who have helped in so many ways to complete this book.

Photographs

Thank you to the photographers and the subjects

- Paul Maggs: Front cover (William, Charlotte and Sarah Maggs)
- Debby Marshall: Figure 4.1 (Renae Roper)
- Paul Maggs: Figure 5.1 (Charlotte Maggs)
- University College London Hospitals: Figure 10.1 (Welcome to our Hospital)
- Dharmini Mistry: Figure 11.1 (Pawly Bear)

Statements at the start of each chapter have been taken from *The common core of skills and knowledge*. This publication is the copyright of the Children's Workforce Development Council (2010) and is available from the National Archive website under the terms of the Open Government Licence, which can be accessed via www.nationalarchives.gov.uk/doc/open-government-licence/version/2.

It is gratefully acknowledged that under © Crown copyright 2012, 'You may re-use this document/publication (not including logos) free of charge in any format or medium, under the terms of the Open Government Licence v2.0. To view this licence visit www.nationalarchives.gov.uk/doc/open-government-licence or write to the Information Policy Team, The National Archives, Kew, Richmond, Surrey, TW9 4DU; or email: psi@nationalarchives.gsi.gov.uk.'

INTRODUCTION

This book has been developed to explore how healthcare professionals can use play and recreation to promote the health and wellbeing of children and young people in a variety of professional contexts and healthcare settings. It aims to promote the use of applied knowledge in practice and the importance of collating evidence to demonstrate how play and recreation can enhance service delivery and provide good 'value for money'.

As this is an edited book, each chapter is self-contained and focuses on a particular theme that is relevant to the delivery of play and recreation. This allows the chapters to be read in any order, according to the reader's own interests or needs.

How the book works

Each chapter follows a similar format. The chapter begins with an introductory overview of the context for the chapter content. This is followed by a set of intended chapter objectives, which are provided as possible cues for engaging with the text. These can also be used to help evaluate, on completion of the chapter, what you may have gained from reading the chapter.

One of the key features of the book is the promotion of effective practice that can be aligned to professional development frameworks within the children and young people's workforce. Two frameworks have been used, one for those working in the National Health Service (NHS) and one for all people who make up the children and young people's workforce.

For those working within the NHS, personal development and review is conducted through the appraisal system based on the *Knowledge and Skills Framework* (KSF), which also forms part of the national terms and conditions of employment for NHS staff (NHS Employers 2010). The original KSF published by the Department of Health (2004) defined 30 areas or dimensions. However, this degree of detail made the KSF time-consuming and cumbersome to use, so a supplement to the original KSF was introduced to simplify and summarize the original six core dimensions (NHS Employers 2010).

The document referred to within this book is *Appraisals and KSF made simple: a practical guide* published by NHS Employers in 2010. Content from this document has been reproduced with kind permission from NHS Employers, and this is gratefully acknowledged.

This book makes reference to the six core dimensions and has picked out some key areas that have been used to tailor chapter content. Each dimension has been divided into four levels, one being the lowest and four the highest. Performance indicators are provided at each level 'describing how the knowledge and skill needs to be applied at that level' (NHS Employers 2010). Some of the most appropriate indicators that match the chapter content have been identified for each chapter. Each dimension also describes what 'behaviours and actions are positive indicators that the knowledge and skills within this dimension are present' (NHS Employers 2010) and, where appropriate, these have also been identified.

Each key area appears as shown in the following example (a description of the differing areas has been added in brackets to this example, taken from Chapter 9):

THE NHS KNOWLEDGE AND SKILLS FRAMEWORK
(professional development framework for those working in the NHS)

Quality (dimension)
- Works as required by relevant trust and professional policies and procedures (indicator at level 1)
- Uses trust resources efficiently and effectively, thinking of cost and environmental issues (indicator at level 1)
- Resources are used effectively (positive indication)

Service improvement (dimension)
- Evaluates own and others' work when needed (indicator at level 2)
- Makes suggestions to improve the service (indicator at level 2)
- Passes on any good ideas to improve services to line manager or appropriate person (indicator at level 1)
- Staff feel they deliver a service to a standard they are personally pleased with (positive indicator)

(NHS Employers 2010)

For all people working with children and young people, including those within the healthcare sector, there is *The common core of skills and knowledge* (CWDC 2010). Although the Children's Workforce Development Council (CWDC) no longer exists and this framework is no longer promoted, it still provides a useful description of 'the skills and knowledge that everyone who works with children and young people [are] expected to have' (CWDC 2010).

The *common core* is made up of six 'areas of expertise' and is presented as a single framework to 'underpin multi-agency and integrated working, professional standards, training and qualifications across the children and young people's workforce' (CWDC 2010: 2).

Each chapter makes reference to the core areas of the and Irena and uses some of the most appropriate numbered descriptors from the three main themes within each core area. These may be part of the introductory descriptors, skills or knowledge.

Again, each appears as follows (a description for the differing areas has been added in brackets to this example, taken from Chapter 9):

THE COMMON CORE OF SKILLS AND KNOWLEDGE
(professional development framework for all those working with children and young people)

Child and young person development (area of expertise)

- Know how to use theory and experience to reflect upon, think about and improve practice... (Knowledge 2.31)
- Understand the impact of technology on children's and young people's lives (Knowledge 2.22)

Multi-agency and integrated working (area of expertise)

- Record, summarise and share information where appropriate, using information and communication technology skills where necessary (Skills 5.7)
- Present facts and judgements objectively (Skills 5.14)
- Be proactive, initiate necessary action and be able to put forward your judgements (Skills 5.11)
- Know about tools, processes and procedures for multi-agency and integrated working, including those for assessment, consent and information sharing (Knowledge 5.28)

(CWDC 2010)

The chapter then moves into an introduction that provides a context for the content of the chapter. The main chapter content will explore why the main theme of the chapter is important and the professional context in which it may take place. Theoretical perspectives are then explored and discussed, suggesting ways in which these can be applied and utilized to enhance professional practice.

Within each chapter, a variety of activities have been suggested that help you to engage with the chapter content, such as case studies or reflective activities to supplement the text. These are not compulsory and the chapter content provides sufficient depth and detail to cover the topic being presented. However, the activities have been designed not only to help explain or clarify specific ideas or topics, but also to 'stretch and challenge the reader' and make the text relevant to the reader's individual interests and professional practice.

For example, to fully understand the explanation of how the KSF has been used within each chapter, it would be advantageous for you to access a copy of *Appraisals and KSF made simple: a practical guide* from NHS Employers (2010) and look at 'Appendix 4: summary descriptions of KSF core dimensions', where the original information was obtained. The activity would begin with a general explanation and then it would set you a task. If necessary, it would direct you to where the additional information can be found, so you can then access that resource or information and use it to complete the activity. If this activity had been set, the second dimension, covering 'service improvement', would have been left blank and you would have been asked to complete the activity using the information provided in the sources given above.

So, the set activity would look like this:

Activity 1

If you work within the NHS, you should be part of an appraisal system that reviews your performance and develops you as a practitioner. This is based on the Knowledge and Skills Framework (KSF) that was introduced by the Department of Health in 2004. A summarized version has been produced that focuses on the six core dimensions. Visit the following website to access a copy of *Appraisals and KSF made simple: a practical guide*, and go to Appendix 4: www.nhsemployers.org/Aboutus/Publications/Documents/Appraisals%20and%20KSF%20made%20simple.pdf.

Look at the dimension covering service improvement and identify which level each of the indicators comes from.

If it is appropriate, suggested answers are provided at the end of the chapter. Each chapter concludes with 'Sources of further information' and 'Further reading' that readers may like to explore as an extension of the chapter content.

Overview of chapter content

Chapter 1 provides a historical overview of the role of play and recreation by exploring the evolution of play, particularly within education, as a precursor for the provision of play and recreation within healthcare settings.

This leads into Chapter 2, which provides worked examples of how play-based activities can be used within healthcare-related practice to help children and young people engage with information relating to what's contained within their bodies and how their bodies work.

Chapter 3 looks at the position of children and young people within the family and society as a whole, promoting reflection and review on how practitioners engage with children and their families to achieve best practice within the health-care sector.

Chapter 4 covers child development and promotes the use of observational methods and data analysis techniques to help identify and evaluate the developmental stage of the individual child or young person. This is particularly important when linked to how health-related issues can impact on children and young people's development.

This leads directly into Chapter 5, which takes observational judgements onto the next stage. It explores play-related theories and identifies how play and recreation can be planned and provided for individual children and young people using age and developmental stage-appropriate provision.

Chapter 6 considers in detail the ways in which resilience can be enhanced for children and young people. It provides an in-depth exploration of the socio-historical perspectives of the experience of being in hospital for children and young people and the effect illness can have on the child and the family as a whole.

Chapter 7 explores how health can be promoted through the use of play and recreation within healthcare settings and the unique position of healthcare professionals to promote health and wellbeing across the age range.

Chapter 8 explores how policy is derived and how it can be used to underpin the provision of play and recreation within healthcare settings. Safeguarding is used as an example of how legislation defines policy development and how this then feeds into practice.

Chapter 9 describes how activities and resources can be investigated to enhance effective provision and explores the investigation processes that are available for those working within the NHS.

With the current focus on child-centred services, Chapter 10 explores the importance of promoting the involvement and participation of children and young people in the design, delivery and evaluation of healthcare services and settings and how this can be done.

Chapter 11 promotes the leadership potential of all people who work within the NHS and how this can be used to promote the importance of play and recreation within healthcare provision.

The final chapter provides examples of how play and recreation are used in practice through a series of case studies from a range of differing healthcare practitioners from a variety of settings. This should draw together the major themes from across the book and show how play and recreation has been used in practice to promote the health and wellbeing of children and young people.

References

CWDC (2010) *The common core of skills and knowledge*, London: Children's Workforce Development Council.

Department of Health (2004) *The NHS Knowledge and Skills Framework. (NHS KSF) and the development review process*, London: Department of Health Publications.

NHS Employers (2010) *Appraisals and KSF made simple: a practical guide*, London: NHS Employers.

1

THE DEVELOPMENT OF PLAY AND RECREATION IN HEALTHCARE SETTINGS

Julia Whitaker, Frances Barbour and Claire Weldon

This chapter will describe the rich and varied history of the role of play and developmentally appropriate activities in the context of those working with children and young people in healthcare settings. Consideration will be given to how these topics link to theoretical and historical perspectives that have influenced our understanding of the need to play.

Chapter objectives

By the end of this chapter you should have an awareness of:

- the historical context of the role of play within healthcare settings;
- the theoretical perspectives that underpin the historical context of the role of play in healthcare settings;
- the benefits of applied, practice-based knowledge within the context of the children and young people's workforce within healthcare settings.

THE NHS KNOWLEDGE AND SKILLS FRAMEWORK

Communication

- Shares and engages thinking with others
  - Accurate information given
  - Appropriate information given

Personal and people development

- Takes responsibility for meeting own development needs
  - People feel they have the knowledge and skills to do their jobs
  - People feel responsible for developing their own expertise

(NHS Employers 2010)

THE COMMON CORE OF SKILLS AND KNOWLEDGE

Effective communication and engagement with children, young people and families

- Summarise situations in the appropriate way for the individual (taking into account factors such as background, age and personality)
- Present genuine choices to children and young people, explaining what has happened or will happen next and what they are consenting to
- Recognise that different people have different interests in a situation and be able to work with them to reach the best and most fair conclusion for the child or young person
- Know when and how to refer to sources of information, advice or support from different agencies or professionals in children's or adult services

Child and young person development

- Encourage children or young people to value their personal experiences and knowledge
- Know how to interact with children and young people in ways that support the development of their ability to think, learn, and become independent

Multi-agency and integrated working

- Understand that others may not have the same understanding of profes-sional terms and may interpret abbreviations and acronyms differently

(CWDC 2010)

Introduction

The need for children to play and have recreation in healthcare settings is not a modern-day concept. It is known that in Victorian times ladies visited children in hospital to read to them and teach them to write. Pictorial images of toys in wards would suggest that in some establishments there was recognition that children needed mental stimulation, as well as physical care, to make a complete recovery. Birrell (1995) supports this idea when he talks about 'play alcoves' that were part of the new Edinburgh Children's Hospital built in 1895, while Barnes (2011) states that around that time in other parts of the United Kingdom, and in line with Florence Nightingale's teaching of the importance of fresh air to aid recovery, open-air schools were introduced and sun verandas with bed space were provided.

Loneliness was a debilitating factor for children separated from their families for long periods of time, and play – as well as ladies reading stories – was seen as one way of addressing this. This loneliness is something that is recalled by former child patients who share their memories of hospital experiences. They recall being away from home with no-one, or anything familiar, to comfort them. Fifty years after her hospital admission in 1954, Jones (in Barnes 2011: 24) describes it as 'the shock of it all'. On visiting, her father was told by a nurse 'well, she hasn't said a word, but she's been a very good girl'. Her parents recall their child just lying there silent and totally withdrawn.

The medical establishment's apparent lack of awareness of the emotional impact of hospitalization on children changed when, in 1952, James and Joyce Robertson, as part of the project *Young children in brief separation* made a short film entitled *A two year old goes to hospital*. The film looked at the problem of admitting a small child who was unable to understand the hospital experience and too young to be away from her mother and everything that was familiar to her.

Theoretical perspectives

The evolution of play in the context of healthcare can be seen to reflect the major landmarks in the way play has been perceived and understood more generally over time.

Jenkinson (2001) provides a helpful historical overview of how our understanding of play has evolved over time. The concept of play as essential to human existence has been recorded since the time of Plato, who recognized a close relationship between creative play and music, dancing and art. Plato described the 'play leap' of all young creatures who are inspired to jump, skip and cry out with the joy of spontaneous movement and self-expression. The physical nature of play is something recognized by present-day movements for outside play and experiential learning – for example forest schools, woodland kindergartens and the Wild Network (2013).

In the nineteenth century the English philosopher Herbert Spencer proposed a theory based on Darwin's *The origin of species* in which play was understood as an outlet for the exuberant energies of childhood. Play was a way to 'let off steam', still a familiar notion in modern times (Spencer 1866).

In the 1890s another philosopher, Karl Groos, compared animal and human play and claimed that play served to train young animals for the roles they would adopt in maturity (Gray 2009). This was an early proposal that 'play is practice for life'. Groos purported that children learn by imitation and therefore need a long and protected childhood in which to practise the wide variety of skills that they will require to be able to function later in life (Groos 1901).

At the start of the twentieth century, Freud's 'psychoanalytic theory' linked behaviour with past experiences and claimed that children's play is likewise determined. Freud observed that children use objects ('toys') to re-create both pleasurable and unpleasant experiences and, in so doing, to gain mastery of events over which in reality they may have little or no control. In play the child becomes active and powerful rather than the passive victim of circumstance.

The child's best loved and most absorbing occupation is play. Perhaps we may say that every child at play behaves like a creative writer, in that he creates a world of his own, or, more truly, he arranges the things of his world and orders it in a new way that pleases him better.

(Freud 1908 [1995])

Melanie Klein and Anna Freud, working in Vienna and London in the 1920s and 1930s, developed Freud's notion of the unconscious and repackaged psychoanalytic theory for children in the form of play therapy. However, it was Virginia Axline and her widely read publication *Dibs, in search of self* (1964) that popularized the understanding of play therapy for a wider audience.

Although play therapy has emerged from differing theories and practices, it unites through 'the central proposition that play transmits and communicates the child's unconscious experiences, desires, thoughts and emotions' (British Association of Play Therapists 2013). As such, this approach is designed to help children 'work through' psychological conflict through the conscious interpretation of their play. This specialized therapeutic approach has had widespread influence on the methods and insights of others working with children.

Donald Winnicott (1988) viewed play as being at the interface between the inner world of the child and external reality. Play was a means by which children could communicate their innermost feelings to another and thereby achieve mastery over them. Again, we see play described as an active agent of change, a language by which the child can safely reveal their innermost thoughts and feelings – to themselves as much as to others.

Case Study 1.1

A boy was diagnosed with type 1 diabetes after a life-threatening collapse at school. His parents were understandably very worried by the diagnosis and impressed upon him how important it was for him to adhere to dietary restrictions and regular medication.

The child resisted attempts to engage him in any discussion about his illness but spent his time in hospital creating and re-creating a racing car circuit on which he organized a race in which one or other driver would crash, die and then be revived. In this way he was trying to make sense of his own experience of near-death and to process his own and his parents' feelings of anxiety.

On the third day, the boy was able to say to the play specialist 'I could have died but I didn't and nobody knows if I'll be so lucky next time.'

Piaget was more interested in the child's intellectual development and the meanings that the child assigns to his or her play. Piaget made a distinction between 'play', which occurs as the child assimilates and internalizes information about the world, and 'imitation', which occurs as the child accommodates and adapts to changing circumstances. Piaget believed that both play and imitation are fundamental to the development of intelligence and social behaviour.

Activity 1.1

The concept of 'imitation' is central to several theories of play. Consider the following:

(a) how a young child plays in imitation of an adult behaviour in the home;
(b) how imitation might be used in a play interaction in the hospital playroom.

Erik Erikson developed psychoanalytic thinking to suggest that a child's play represents a metaphor for his or her life and offers a window on any anxieties and pre-occupations – both good and bad. Erikson also believed that children's play could reveal something of their future selves in the sense that it is creative as well as re-creative of experience. Through play, a child will show how he or she wants things to change or become, including his or her perception of him- or herself (Erikson 1963).

In the 1920s Rudolf Steiner had also written of play as a signpost towards the nature of the child in the future:

> In playing, children show the same form as they will when they find their way into life. Children who play slowly will also be slow at the age of twenty and think slowly about all their experiences. Children who are superficial in play will be superficial later. Children who say that they want to break open their toys to see what they look like inside will later become philosophers. That is the kind of thinking that overcomes the problems of life. In play you can certainly do very much.
>
> *(Steiner 1920: 95)*

The early theorists made attempts to understand the meaning of play from an individualistic perspective, but as the twentieth century unfolded, greater emphasis was placed on the social aspects of play and the function it serves in supporting the child's relationships with others and with the wider world. Smilansky (1990) coined the term 'sociodramatic play' to describe the role-playing that children incorporate into their games. Sociodramatic play begins as imitation of adult interactions, but is combined with make-believe which allows children to develop imaginary scenarios and to create their own realities. Smilansky found that opportunities for sociodramatic play, free from adult interference, promoted social integration and competence as flexible and adaptive participants in the social community.

Activity 1.2

Consider the following:

(a) how healthcare institutions can sometimes inhibit social interaction between children;
(b) how healthcare practitioners could create and allow opportunities for social play.

The researchers Curry and Arnaud (1984) looked at sociodramatic play from a cross-cultural perspective and found common themes across different cultural traditions, despite variations in play style and content. Children universally play-out family relationships, domestic scenarios, medical interactions and aggressive or frightening themes such as fighting or monsters. Play is one universal element of healthcare provision for children, capable of transcending barriers of language, gender and tradition. It is accessible to all regardless of age or ability and can be a force for unity.

Case Study 1.2

Two children are playing together at being nurses in the hospital playroom. They have put on aprons and gloves and are trying to encourage the dolls to take their medicine.
Child A coaxes, with promises of sweets and being able to go home early.
Child B commands 'Swallow! Don't vomit or I will be very angry.'
The children share a common play theme, albeit using different play styles. Their individual contributions to the game reflect their different experiences of being parented (imitation) but they share a level of reality which is inclusive and respectful of this difference.

It is now widely accepted that play is not only an essential component of human experience as expressed by Schiller (2012) in an essay dated 1795, but that it is crucial to the child's all-round development. Play is how children learn about themselves and about the world. It is the way in which they make a connection with others and find their place in society. Play may reflect the past experiences that have shaped the individual, but also serves to point towards the future that the child might create for themselves. Western governments have taken on board the evidence that play is a medium to be recognized and valued as key to a child's development and growth. Parents are encouraged to play with their children from infancy and play is a central feature of early years and school curriculums.

Any consideration of the theoretical understanding of play cannot ignore the role of technology in children's play in the twenty-first century. Computer games in all their forms have, in many ways, usurped the place of traditional games and the consequences of this fact have already begun to emerge. In Western societies we face the growing problem of childhood obesity, which to a large extent is due to the passive nature of leisure dominated by electronic media. Greater numbers of children are being diagnosed and medicated for attention deficit problems and the incidence of mental health problems among the young are the highest ever recorded (Public Health England 2013). There is a growing movement of interested parties (e.g. International Association for the Child's Right to Play; Alliance for Childhood) who are determined to address this trend by persuading those with social influence to restore childhood as a protected time with play at its heart.

Play in education

When Robert Owen established the first nursery provision for the young children of millworkers in New Lanark, Scotland in 1816 he insisted that this should involve no formal teaching but be a purely playful experience.

The development of play in hospital and other healthcare settings needs to be placed in the context of the development of play in education and governmental approaches to the early years as embodied in the current Early Years Framework. In England, the Early Years Foundation Stage (EYFS) is the statutory framework that sets the standards that all early years providers must meet to ensure that children learn and develop well and are kept healthy and safe (Department for Education 2012). It promotes teaching and learning to ensure children are ready for school and gives children the broad range of knowledge and skills that provide the right foundation for good future progress through school and life. Equivalent standards apply in the Scottish *Early Years Framework, Curriculum for Excellence* and in the Welsh *Foundation Phase.*

While play has long been recognized as the starting point for early learning, formal state education was initially typically characterized by an absence of play and a focus on rote learning under the direct instruction of the teacher. Following the *Education Act of 1870*, and the introduction of compulsory elementary education ten years later, very young children were admitted to schools along with their older siblings in order to protect them from the risks associated with 'slum life'. The formal teaching methods practised were evidently unsuitable for young minds and it was officially recognized that under-fives required a different approach.

Early education pioneers who shared Owen's humanitarian values, the Macmillan sisters, established an open-air nursery in 1911 in South London, with the aim of promoting the health and wellbeing of the children of working class families. The nursery afforded opportunities for free play in the fresh air and Margaret McMillan became the first president of the Nursery School Association (now the British Association for Early Childhood Education). McMillan's methods were replicated in open-air provision during the early twentieth century and have found renewed popularity in the forest school movement and the more widespread appreciation of outdoor play and learning (Forest Research 2013).

Activity 1.3

Most healthcare providers are now aware of the importance of an outdoor space designed with children in mind and new-build hospitals have incorporated creative outdoor play areas such as roof gardens and terraces.

Consider the provision of outdoor play opportunities in the healthcare setting in which you work. Do you consider them conducive to healthy play and learning in the fresh air?

There may be significant differences in the approaches of the pioneers of early childhood education, but a common principle is that the early years curriculum and practice methods must be adaptable to the changing needs, abilities and interests of the child (Elkind 2007). Healthcare practitioners, likewise, need to ensure that they approach each child as an individual and are not biased by normative expectations.

This principle of 'individualism' was embodied in the kindergarten movement, developed by Friedrich Froebel (1782–1852) and attributed as being the first early childhood curriculum to be widely adopted in both Europe and abroad.

Prior to Froebel's kindergarten, children below the age of seven did not attend school in Europe. It was believed that young children did not have the ability to focus or to develop cognitive and emotional skills before this age. However, Froebel expressed his own beliefs about the importance of early education, linking the 'eruption of consciousness' to when learning begins. Froebel labelled his approach to education as 'self-activity'. This idea allows the child to be led by his or her own interests and to freely explore them. Froebel called play 'the work of the child' and acknowledged its place as key to the educational process.

Rudolf Steiner (1861–1925) also advocated child-led free play both in and out of doors. In the Steiner kindergarten there is no adult interference in play and neither is it planned beforehand nor dictated by educational goals. Steiner believed that children uncover their own learning in play and that the imagination is essential for the development of intellectual concepts and encourages creativity and flexibility later on.

The kindergarten movement was propelled by the industrial revolution and the introduction of women into the factory labour force, and subsequently by the need for mothers to replace male workers who had been enlisted to fight in the First and Second World Wars.

Free play, which was integral to an early years curriculum with the child at the centre, had a powerful influence on American education too, through the work of John Dewey (1859–1952). His 'Lab School' trained teachers to observe and follow children's natural inclinations and interests rather than directing them. Evidence accrued that important skills such as problem solving, communication and mathematical concepts developed as children were allowed to move freely in and out of the classroom and to explore their surroundings. Throughout the process children and teachers became learners together.

Activity 1.4

The hospital environment is not typically one that allows free movement to children, for obvious reasons of health and safety. However, a creative play specialist can design a play space that allows for optimum flow between activities and includes opportunities for young patients to choose between different types of play.

Consider how you might re-arrange a play space in your own work environment to allow children freedom in their choice of play.

Maria Montessori's (1870–1952) approach to early education was also widely adopted both in Europe and abroad. Her emphasis was less on learning through exploratory play, but rather on the teaching of essential skills by breaking them down into their constituent movements and actions. Children were encouraged to learn independently but in a carefully constructed environment using purposeful exercises and equipment. In a Montessori nursery, young children will learn to write by first tracing sandpaper letters with their fingers and later with chalk or pencil. Today, mainstream education provision has adopted key aspects of Montessori's methods, based on her belief that early education can be beneficial to society as a whole. However it was not until after the Second World War that early childhood education was truly accepted as crucial to development.

Vygotsky (1896–1934) differed from those who believed that children's development occurs spontaneously (Froebel, Steiner, Dewey) and also from those who claimed that teaching could alter the process of development regardless of the child's age or ability. Vygotsky's theory was that learning can encourage development if it occurs within a 'zone of proximal development' (ZPD), at the point when the child is on the brink of acquiring new skills and concepts. If our expectations of a child lie outside their proximal zone, then even the most strenuous teaching methods may fail to achieve results. Vygotsky recognized that the kind of support a child needs in order to develop new skills and concepts within their ZPD will differ with the child's age. For example, imaginary play with a pre-schooler could offer the same prospect for learning as direct instruction for an older child. Children are seen as active participants in their own learning, through their interactions with others and with their social environment. Vygotsky believed that children were not merely imitators, but co-constructors of their future knowledge, skills and attitudes:

A child's greatest achievements are possible in play, achievements that will tomorrow become her basic level of real action and morality.

(Vygotsky 1978: 100)

Activity 1.5

Consider the following and then give examples of how you might prepare a child at different ages for an event or procedure familiar to you:

(a) A play specialist preparing a young child for the taking of a blood sample might invent a little play or puppet show which involves a character undergoing the test.
(b) For an older child, they may describe the procedure in words, showing the relevant equipment to support their description.
(c) For a young person, words alone may be sufficient.

The play specialist will base their 'teaching' method on their observations of the child or young person at play and their assessment of their developmental stage.

The case for play as an obvious starting point for education is convincing, although not without its critics. Research evidence has shown that free play does not maximize cognitive development – but should this be regarded as a goal of early childhood? Sylva *et al.* (1980) studied how both children and adults spend their time during free play sessions and found that these were characterized by the simple repetition of activities and a lack of challenging diversions. Meadows and Cashdan (1988), in a similar investigation, reported that during free play children did not persist at tasks and that communication between adult and child was limited. Meadows and Cashdan concluded that a high level of adult–child interaction during play is necessary to optimize children's learning.

Inequalities in educational outcomes have prompted modern governments to look at ways of targeting disadvantaged pre-school children for enhanced learning opportunities. The Head Start programme launched in the United States in the 1960s for children of low-income families represents a modern trend in governmental involvement in setting the early years agenda. Head Start became a model for similar programmes worldwide – including Sure Start, established in the United Kingdom in 1998, which endeavoured to reduce the impact of child poverty by 'enhancing the social and cognitive development of children through provision of educational, health, nutritional, social and other services' (Weigel 2011). This has now been embraced as part of a move towards 'early intervention', although implementation is still seen as problematic (Action for Children 2013).

While investment in such programmes may be well-intended, an unintended consequence is that it affords the impression that education is a race, and the sooner it is started, the earlier and better the finish. The exclusive focus on cognitive development (rather than any other aspect) suggests that educational success is more important than any other outcome measure. There is an obvious dissonance between the child-centred approach to learning, advocated by the pioneers of early education, and an early start to formal education. In countries that have a long history of pre-school education, such as the Scandinavian countries, the Netherlands and Italy, a child-centred approach is the norm. Play is accepted as the starting point for learning and there is also an emphasis on outdoor play in the natural environment. However, in countries with a more competitive and test-driven education system (such as the United States, United Kingdom and Japan), many children are expected to start formal education at an early age. It is worth noting that in a league table of child wellbeing in 29 of the world's most advanced economies, the Netherlands comes top and the Scandinavian countries fill the remaining top five places, while the United Kingdom stands in sixteenth place and the United States at number 26 (Unicef United Kingdom 2013).

There are many challenges to the concept of a long and protected early childhood devoted to play, as imagined by the pioneers of early education. Changes in family structure and lifestyle, statutory intervention in early years care and education and the undeniable impact of electronic media have changed the landscape in which our youngest citizens grow and develop. However, the human drive to play for pleasure and learning remains undiminished.

A historical perspective of play in healthcare settings

A holistic approach to healthcare will recognize that any medical episode is usually but a brief interlude in the child's life and the need for consistency across settings cannot be overemphasized. When healthcare practitioners can work in partnership with education and care providers, the child will find security and comfort in what is familiar to them.

Case Study 1.3

A four-year-old child was due to be admitted for cardiac surgery, and her parents met with the play specialist to discuss how best to prepare her for her hospital admission.

The play specialist asked about the child's developmental progress and tailored her advice and guidance based on what she learned about the child and her interests. With the parents' consent, the play specialist liaised with the child's nursery teacher and together they devised an activity that the teacher could do with the whole class to help both the young patient and her classmates prepare for her hospital stay. The teacher's own observations and opinions enhanced information obtained from the parental interview and ensured that healthcare staff were able to adapt their actions and interventions to the individual needs of the child.

The benefits of play to the wellbeing and health of the child are irrefutable and are covered in detail within Chapter 7. Rogers *et al.* (2009) have summarized the benefits as follows:

- Happiness – plenty of time for play in childhood is linked to happiness in adulthood.
- Physical activity – active play facilitates children's development of spatial abilities and an understanding of the world through the senses and movement.
- Cognitive skills – there is a close link between play and cognitive development.
- Social and emotional learning – make-believe play is related to better overall emotional health and social functioning.

As noted above, *A two year old goes to hospital* was instrumental in changing attitudes to how children and their families were cared for in healthcare settings. However, this change took time. When the film was first shown at the Royal Society of Medicine, in November 1952, many paediatricians found it difficult to accept that the children in their wards were not happy. In 1957 Sir Harry Platt and members of the Committee on the Welfare of Children in Hospital were shown the film. Two years later, the Platt Report was published and, for the first time, the way children were looked after in hospital was highlighted to both medical staff and, perhaps more importantly, the general public (Robertson 1970). The Platt Report made 55 recommendations for the non-medical care of children. One recommendation recognized that children needed to be kept happy and have interesting things to do. It was the public, in particular mothers, who started campaigning to improve conditions for sick children. A group was formed called 'Mother Care for Children in Hospital', which later became known as the National Association for the Welfare of Children in Hospital (NAWCH). The organization is now known as Action for Sick Children and Action for Sick Children Scotland.

Peg Belson, a founder member of NAWCH, worked alongside the National Association of Health Play Staff (NAHPS) to raise awareness of the importance of play in hospital. Belson (cited in Barnes 2011) states that those caring for sick children considered it 'natural' for children to cry in hospital and felt that children soon forgot about their experience. A good ward routine was seen to be paramount in the smooth running of a hospital and there were genuine concerns about the risk of cross-infection. Little consideration was given to the emotional effect of separation, especially on the young child. The work undertaken by NAWCH was instrumental in making changes to the visiting rights of children and parents, when in 1966 discussion in the House of Commons established a clear definition of visiting arrangements, stating that fixed visiting hours had to be abandoned and a more flexible approach adopted.

The work of these organizations and individuals is reflected in our practice today. Without this rich history and inspiration, children's and young people's healthcare would be a lot poorer. Clearly, much is still being done to develop our

TABLE 1.1 Timeline of the development of play in hospital

The innovative work carried out in 1963 by Susan Harvey, a Save the Children Fund advisor, led to the first Hospital Play Worker, Gabi Marston, being employed at the Brook Hospital, London. Susan Harvey is credited with being the founder member of play in hospital.

1972 The Department of Health and Social Security commissioned an expert group on Play in Hospital, which made recommendations for the employment of play staff on children's wards. Their report was published in 1976.

1973 Under the guidance of Susan Harvey, Gabi Marston and Dr Hugh Jolly, the first training course for Hospital Play Specialists was set up at Chiswick College. The course moved to Southwark College in 1978 and was the forerunner of today's hospital play specialist training.

1975 The National Association of Hospital Play Staff (NAHPS) was set up and comprised 28 play staff and ten other professional people, including nurses, doctors and social workers.

1985 The Hospital Play Staff Examination Board (HPSEB) was set up with the aid of a grant from the Department of Health, as a totally independent educational trust with charitable status, to separate the training course from the support function of the professional association NAHPS.

1998 The Hospital Play Staff Education Trust (HPSET) ratified a policy on re-registration for Hospital Play Specialists (HPS).

2000 Re-registration was introduced and has provided the qualified play specialist with the opportunity to demonstrate evidence of continuing professional development (CPD) based on the updating of knowledge and skills.

2003 The Department of Health published the National Service Framework for Children, Young People and Maternity Services. The standard for hospital services makes reference to the need for play in hospital and the therapeutic purpose of play as part of the child's care plan. The document recommends that all children staying in hospital have daily access to a play specialist.

2004 Edexcel and HPSET introduced a new Level 4 qualification – A Professional Diploma in Specialised Play for Sick Children and Young People – accredited at Level 4 on the National Qualification Framework.

2008 Following extensive consultation, HPSET approved the proposal that the current programme of study should be a Foundation Degree, with entry to the professional register at Level 5. Pilot programmes were validated by Thames Valley University (now the University of West London) to commence in September 2010 at Bolton College and Stanmore College.

The Foundation Degree in 'Healthcare Play Specialism' (FdA HPS) is recognized as the newest requirement for application for professional registration with HPSET and a licence to practice as a registered play specialist. The qualification and professional registration together form the recognized qualification and standard for work in the NHS and many community healthcare settings.

2011 All hospital play specialists registered with HPSET were invited to re-register every two years from the date of initial registration, or from the expiry date of the current period of training.

2012 Peg Belson, the Patron of NAHPS and founder member of the National Association for the Welfare of Children in Hospital (NAWCH), died.

Reproduced with kind permission from the National Association of Health Play Specialists (2013).

knowledge, skills and understanding. As health practitioners, it is our responsibility to ensure that children and young people have equal access to suitable play and recreational activities, led by appropriately trained people, while affording them the opportunity to benefit fully from their experiences.

Suggested answers to activity questions

Activity 1.1

(a) A child at home may imitate a parent talking on the phone or making a cup of tea.
(b) A child in hospital may imitate a doctor or nurse writing notes, or use a doll's pram to represent a hospital trolley taking a patient to X-ray.

Activity 1.2

(a) Children nursed in individual rooms or in isolation will have little or no contact with peers.
Meals may be served at the bedside.
Infection control policies may prohibit the sharing of toys.
(b) Play specialists work to encourage social opportunities wherever possible, with group sessions in the playroom, storytelling and puppet shows. Where children are nursed individually, they can still send messages and pictures between each other, especially with the advance of interactive technology. The play specialist can invite a number of children to contribute individually to a joint project, such as a collage or other artistic endeavour.

Activity 1.3

The benefits of outdoor play are well documented and the Statutory Framework for the EYFS (Department of Health 2012) states that 'Providers must provide access to an outdoor play area or, if that is not possible, ensure that outdoor activities are planned and taken on a daily basis (unless circumstances make this inappropriate, for example unsafe weather conditions).' This would suggest that opportunities for outdoor play should be incorporated into routines within healthcare settings wherever possible. See Chapter 7 for further information relating to health and wellbeing and the outdoors.

Activity 1.4

A play space needs to accommodate children's holistic needs with equal attention given to their physical, intellectual, social and emotional development. A successful play space will be an organic space that reflects the changing needs and moods of the user group, offering a balance between familiarity and novelty:

- A well designed play area will provide opportunities for free movement for a wide range of physical abilities. Is there somewhere to hide? Somewhere to climb? Something to crawl through?
- The furnishings need to allow for children to play together and for parents to play with their children.
- There also needs to be a quiet, cosy corner where a child can be alone yet feel safe and secure.
- Are cupboards and toy boxes labelled in a way that children can find their way around the resources without adult help? Is there enough to offer sufficient choice but not so much that it is overwhelming?

Activity 1.5 (possible examples)

(a) (Under seven years)

'Tufty the squirrel puppet has a sore tail and his Mummy cannot work out why. She's looked at it, sniffed it, kissed it, but it's still sore so she takes Tufty to see Dr Brown (owl puppet)....'

(b) (Over seven years)

'A doctor is a bit like a detective when he/she is trying to work out what's causing someone's problem and how to solve it. The doctor has to search for clues and one of the best clues is to be found in a person's blood....'

(c) (Over 12)

'I will talk you through the different steps involved in having a blood test and you can ask me about anything you don't understand....'

Sources of further information

Action for Sick Children: www.actionforsickchildren.org.uk
Action for Sick Children Scotland: www.ascscotland.org.uk
Alliance for Childhood: www.allianceforchildhood.org.uk
European Association for Children in Hospital (EACH): www.each-for-sick-children.org
Fair Play for Children: www.fairplayforchildren.org
International Play Association: http://ipaworld.org

References

Action for Children (2013) *Early intervention: where now for local authorities*, Watford: Action for Children.

Axline, V. (1964) *Dibs in search of self: personality development in play therapy.* Boston, MA: Houghton Mifflin.

Barnes, P.A. (ed.) (2011) *Celebration of a transformation: 50 years of action for sick children*, Stockport: Action for Sick Children.

Birrell, G. (1995) *A most perfect hospital: the centenary of the Royal Hospital for Sick Children, Edinburgh*, Edinburgh: Metro Press.

British Association of Play Therapists (2013) *A history of play therapy*, Online. Available: www.bapt.info/historyofpt.htm (accessed 2 December 2013).

Curry, N.E. and Arnaud, S.H. (1984) Play in developmental pre-school settings, In: Yawkey, T. and Pelligrini, A. (eds), *Child's play: developmental and applied*, Hillsdale, NJ: Lawrence Erlbaum Associates.

CWDC (Children's Workforce Development Council) (2010) *The common core of skills and knowledge*, Leeds: Children's Workforce Development Council.

Department for Education (2012) *Statutory framework for the early years foundation stage 2012*, Cheshire: Department for Education.

Elkind, D. (2007) *The power of play: how spontaneous, imaginative activities lead to happier, healthier children – learning what comes naturally*, Cambridge, MA: Da Capo Lifelong.

Erikson, E.H. (1963) *Childhood and society*, New York: Norton.

Forest Research (2013) *Forest School in England and Wales and its impact on young children*, Online. Available: www.forestry.gov.uk/fr/infd-5z3jvz (accessed 2 December 2013).

Freud, S. (1995) *The Freud reader*, Gay, P. (ed.), New York: W.W. Norton.

Gray, P. (2009) *The Value of Play IV: Nature's Way of Teaching Us New Skills*. Online. Available: www.psychologytoday.com/blog/freedom-learn/200901/the-value-play-iv-nature-s-way-teaching-us-new-skills (accessed 2 December 2013).

Groos, K. (1901) *The play of man*, New York: Appleton.

Jenkinson, S. (2001) *The genius of play: celebrating the spirit of childhood*, Stroud: Hawthorn Press.

Meadows, S. and Cashdan, A. (1988) *Helping children learn: contributions to a cognitive curriculum*, London: David Fulton Publishers.

National Association of Health Play Specialists (2013) *National Association of Hospital Play staff milestones*, Online. Available: http://nahps.org.uk/index.php?page=history (accessed 2 December 2013).

NHS Employers (2010) *Appraisals and KSF made simple: a practical guide*, London: NHS Employers.

Public Health England (2013) *How healthy behaviour supports children's wellbeing*, London: PHE Publications.

Robertson, J. (1970) *Young children in hospital*, 2nd edn, London: Tavistock Publications.

Rogers, S., Pelletier, C. and Clark, A. (2009) *Play and outcomes for children and young people: literature review to inform the national evaluation of play pathfinders and play builders*, DCSF.

Schiller, F. (2012) *On the aesthetic education of man*, Mineola, NY: Dover Publications.

Smilansky, S. (1990) *Sociodramatic play: its relevance to behaviour and achievement in school, in children's play and learning – perspectives and policy implications*, New York: Teachers College Press.

Spencer, H. (1866) *Education: intellectual, moral and physical*, A.L. Burt Company.

Steiner, R. (1920) *Faculty meetings with Rudolf Steiner, Volume 1*, New York: Anthroposophic Press.

Sylva, K., Roy, C. and McIntyre, G. (1980) *Child watching at playgroup and nursery school*, London: Grant McIntyre.

Unicef United Kingdom (2013) *Report card 11: child well-being in rich countries – a comparative overview*, Florence: Unicef UK.

Vygotsky, L.S. (1978) *Mind in society: the development of higher psychological processes*, Cambridge, MA: Harvard University Press.

Weigel, M. (2011, 11 August) *Head Start impact: Department of Health and Human Services report*. Online. Available: http://journalistsresource.org/studies/government/civil-rights/head-start-study/# (accessed 2 December 2013).

Wild Network (2013) *Project Wild Thing*. Online. Available: http://projectwildthing.com/film (accessed 2 December 2013).

Winnicott, D.W. (1988) *Playing and reality*, London: Penguin.

2

ANATOMY AND PHYSIOLOGY

Applied knowledge in practice

Alison Tonkin

This chapter will demonstrate how knowledge of anatomy and physiology can be applied in practice, particularly with regard to the preparation of children and young people for medical interventions and investigations. It will also show how play techniques and materials can be used to enhance the process.

Chapter objectives

By the end of this chapter you should have an awareness of:

- the link between anatomy and physiology and medical conditions;
- how to link knowledge of anatomy and physiology to medical investigations;
- the theoretical perspectives that underpin how information may be presented;
- how consideration of the age and developmental stage of children and young people can enhance the sharing of anatomical and physiological knowledge;
- the benefits of applied, practice-based knowledge when working within the multidisciplinary team.

THE NHS KNOWLEDGE AND SKILLS FRAMEWORK

Communication

- Shares and engages thinking with others
  - Accurate information given
  - Appropriate information given

Personal and people development

- Takes responsibility for meeting own development needs
  - People feel they have the knowledge and skills to do their jobs
  - People take responsibility for developing their own expertise

(NHS Employers 2010)

THE COMMON CORE OF SKILLS AND KNOWLEDGE

Effective communication and engagement with children, young people and families

- Summarise situations in the appropriate way for the individual (taking into account factors such as background, age and personality)
- Present genuine choices to children and young people, explaining what has happened or will happen next and what they are consenting to
- Recognise that different people have different interests in a situation and be able to work with them to reach the best and most fair conclusion for the child or young person
- Know when and how to refer to sources of information, advice or support from different agencies or professionals in children's or adult services

Child and young person development

- Encourage children or young people to value their personal experiences and knowledge
- Know how to interact with children and young people in ways that support the development of their ability to think, learn and become independent

Multi-agency and integrated working

- Understand that others may not have the same understanding of professional terms and may interpret abbreviations and acronyms differently

(CWDC 2010)

Introduction

Anatomy is the study of the body and how the various parts that make up the body are arranged, while physiology describes how the living body actually works. As a practitioner working within the healthcare sector, you will not necessarily be expected to have a deep understanding of how the human body works or remember technical details of all the major body systems and their component parts. However, you will be expected to know where detailed information can be found and how this can be linked to the provision of care and the promotion of wellbeing for the children and young people you meet within your professional practice (Agenda for Change Project Team 2004). There are a range of excellent textbooks and web-based resources that explore and describe the anatomy and physiology of the human body. This chapter seeks to provide an overview of how knowledge of anatomy and physiology gained from other sources can be applied in practice.

Knowledge can be defined as an 'understanding of or information about a subject which has been obtained by experience or study' (Cambridge Dictionary Online

2013a). However, this definition is contentious, as according to Chapman (2009) when describing the work of Bloom (1956), knowledge and understanding represent different levels of learning. The application of knowledge is a higher-level cognitive skill and, according to Bloom (1956), the application of knowledge requires understanding, not just comprehension. However, this is not always the case. For example, when driving a car you know that when you turn the ignition key, hopefully, the engine will start, but you are not required to understand how turning the key starts the engine – you just know that it does! These distinctions between knowledge, understanding and application are important as they have practical implications for the way in which information should be presented, according to who needs that information and under what circumstances the information is given. This will be discussed in more detail later in the chapter.

Why is knowledge of anatomy and physiology important?

For practitioners to perform their job role with confidence in a competent manner, knowledge of anatomy and physiology provides a support structure that allows information to be put into context. When working with children and young people, there will be times when providing an explanation of how the body works is a key part of the preparation for a procedure. You may be required to facilitate cooperation by a young child for a medical investigation or promote compliance by a young person as part of a treatment regime. However, there will also be times when you interact and share information with members of the multidisciplinary team, some of whom will use technical language and medical terminology that requires knowledge of body systems and how they work.

Naive concepts that have been built up from childhood often 'inform' the provision of health-related information, resulting in inaccurate information being offered. When Ofsted (2004) was commissioned to investigate young children's education of food and nutrition, all pre-school settings demonstrated good evidence of effective practice, whereas the majority of schools did not. Within the pre-school settings, there were numerous factors that were identified, but one significant factor was that 'the knowledge of those engaged in teaching nutrition and developing children's understanding about food and health was accurate, based on informed and current nutritional advice, and free from bias' (Ofsted 2004: 4). In contrast, the poor results obtained within the majority of schools were attributed, in part, to teachers lacking 'sufficient accurate and up-to-date nutrition knowledge, and the confidence and competence they needed to teach children effectively' (Ofsted 2004: 5). This demonstrates the importance of appropriate knowledge for building professional confidence and the link to the effective provision of accurate information that is fit for purpose.

For many adults, knowledge of the body and how it works is limited, even when they have a medical condition that necessitates some understanding of how their body functions (Schmidt 2001). This is not helped when many of the words used to describe various organs and body systems still rely on the original Greek and Latin roots for anatomical structures (Rae-Dupree and DuPree 2007). This means that intuitive awareness of body parts and their functioning is not sufficient, particularly when dealing with members of the multidisciplinary team who may have studied anatomy and physiology for many years!

Linking anatomy and physiology to medical conditions

A condition is defined as 'the particular state that something or someone is in' (Cambridge Dictionary Online 2013b), so a medical condition is the state that someone is in due to an illness or injury.

To appreciate the potential effects an illness or injury may have on the body, a good knowledge of how the body functions under normal circumstances is essential. When linked to knowledge of how medical names and conditions have been 'built' through a systematic process using roots, prefixes and suffixes, medical terminology linked to the functioning of the body can be broken down into a more manageable and logical process.

For example, a key function of the urinary system is the removal of excess fluid from the body. This is performed by the kidneys and the functioning unit of the kidney is the nephron. The name 'nephron' derives from the Greek word root 'neprh', which means kidney. When the kidneys do not function effectively, excess fluid may collect in the body tissue, causing the tissue to swell, which is known as oedema. Therefore, when a child presents with oedema and is diagnosed with a condition such as nephrotic syndrome, you can link the root of the diagnosis to the kidney (*nephr*) making the likely origin of the oedema the failure of the kidneys to remove excess fluid from the body. This demonstrates the value of knowing how the names of medical terms and conditions have originated, allowing links to be made between medical conditions, body components and their related functions.

Medical terminology is usually made up of a combination of a:

- prefix – added to the beginning of a word to make a new word;
- root – origin;
- suffix – added to the end of a word to make a new word.

A prefix can be placed before a suffix and an 'o' is often used as a link between the two, e.g. angiography is an imaging technique that looks inside blood vessels, so an *angiogram* is the picture of the blood vessels that is produced, i.e. *angi* (vessel) – *o* – *gram* (record or picture).

Knowledge of medical roots, prefixes and suffixes and how they link together makes the vast array of medical terms and conditions far less inhibiting (Table 2.1).

The classical origin of the root is also important and this can sometimes lead to confusion (Table 2.2).

For example, an X-ray image of the breast is known as a *mammogram*, while removal of the breast is known as a *mast*ectomy. Both terms relate to the breast but have different origins.

Positional information, size and shape can also be linked to general conditions using combinations of prefixes and roots (Table 2.3).

TABLE 2.1 Examples of prefixes, suffixes and roots relating to body components/functions

Prefixes	Suffixes	Roots
Aden – gland	Algia – pain	Enter – intestine
Bronch – air passage	Gram – record or picture	Gastro – stomach
Cardi – heart	Itis – inflammation	Odont – tooth
Cyst – urinary bladder	Lith – stone	Oste – bone
Mening – membrane	Oma – tumour	Phleb – vein
Rect – rectum	Rhoea – flowing or discharge	Steth – chest

TABLE 2.2 Examples of Greek and Latin roots for body components

Body component	Greek root	Latin root
Kidney	Nephr-	Ren-
Breast	Mast-	Mamm-
Lungs	Pneumon-	Pulmon-
Rib	Pleur-	Cost-
Brain	Encephal-	Cerebr-

TABLE 2.3 Examples of Greek and Latin prefixes and roots combined to identify medical conditions

Prefix	Root	Medical condition
Dys – bad	Pepsia – digestion	Dyspepsia – impaired digestion
Endo – inner	Metr – uterus	Endometrium – inner lining of the uterus
Epi – over or above	Derm – skin	Epidermis – outer layer of the skin
Tachy – fast	Cardi – heart	Tachycardia – fast heartbeat
Intra – within, inside	Ocul – eye	Intraocular pressure – inside the eye

Activity 2.1

Without looking in a medical dictionary, work out what the following medical terms mean:

phlebitis, nephrolith, gastroenteritis, meningioma, nephralgia, bronchorrhoea

Making the link to medical investigations

A similar process can be undertaken when linking body components and systems to medical investigations and surgical techniques (Table 2.4).

TABLE 2.4 Examples of Greek and Latin prefixes and suffixes used to name medical procedures

Prefixes	Suffixes
Arthr – joint	ology – the study of
Neur – nervous system	ectomy – surgical removal
Lobo – related to a lobe	opsy – looking at
Lapar – abdominal cavity	oscopy – looking at with a scope
Hyster – uterus	otomy – surgical incision
Hist – tissue	plasty – modify or reshape
Myo – muscle	stomy – creating a hole

Medical personnel and departments can also be identified using a similar classification system. As identified above, '*ology*' is the study of a subject and an '*ologist*' is someone who studies that subject. For example, a histologist studies the function and composition of body tissues within a histology department, while a cardiologist studies the heart in the cardiology department. However, this is not always straightforward, i.e. a nephrologist studies the kidney, but within a hospital the urinary system as a whole defines the department, which is often known as Urology or, retaining its Latin root, the Renal Unit.

Activity 2.2

Without looking in a medical dictionary, identify the following medical investigations, procedures and departments:

arthroplasty, hysterectomy, orthodontics, laparoscopy, colostomy, histology, myotomy, cardiology, nephrectomy, cystogram, neurology, cystoscopy, arthroscopy

This knowledge should allow you to identify what body component or system is being referred to and what type of investigation or procedure is being considered. From here, you can find out more specific information about the individual procedure, including preparation and post-procedural effects that will determine how you approach the task ahead.

Theoretical perspectives

According to the Agenda for Change Project Team (2004: 5), 'the NHS KSF is about "the application" of knowledge and skills – not about the specific knowledge and skills that individuals need to possess … it does "not" describe the exact knowledge and skills that people need to develop'.

As a healthcare practitioner, there is no formal requirement for you to engage in training or development activities relating to anatomy and physiology unless, of course, it is part of professional training. However, there will be occasions when such knowledge will enhance your own professional practice and therefore the onus is on you as a competent practitioner to ensure you have sufficient knowledge to carry out your job role effectively (NHS Employers 2010).

Activity 2.3

Read the indicators (from the NHS KSF) for 'HWB1/Level 2: Plan, develop and implement approaches to promote health and wellbeing and prevent adverse effects on health and wellbeing' (Agenda for Change Project Team 2004: 89).

Identify an occasion when you have used knowledge of how the body works to encourage a child to comply with a treatment regime to prevent adverse effects due to their medical condition.

Reflect on how your approach may change if you were required to use the same knowledge for a young person suffering from a similar condition.

Limited research has been identified that specifically links children's awareness of what lies inside their bodies to medical procedures. Therefore, sources of evidence are often dated, but their content is still relevant today. Schmidt (2001) presented a review of studies published between 1935 and 2000 that looked at children's body knowledge, focusing on the lungs and their functions. The review suggested that children under the age of nine years do not have an accurate understanding of how their lungs function, particularly the flow of inspired and expired air. This meant they could have difficulty using a peak flow meter effectively as part of the self-management of conditions such as asthma (Schmidt 2001).

It should be noted that knowledge acquisition does not necessarily require understanding for the experience to be useful (de Boo 2001). However, children's understanding of procedures can be enhanced by providing appropriate information prior to a procedure being undertaken (Jun Tai 2008). Therefore, providing health-related information not only enhances active participation in the decision-making process, but may also reduce the fear of pain related to a particular experience (Jun Tai 2008).

According to Gaudion (1997: 14) 'health teaching is inseparable from advocacy and from children's rights' and therefore, the provision of anatomical and physiological information is essential if children and young people are to be active participants in the decision-making process. Respect for autonomy is considered to be the most important ethical principle (Baines 2008) and the need to involve children and young people in decisions about their care is now advocated whenever possible (NHS Choices 2011). The way information is presented is important and it needs to be tailored to the individual. For example, the children's version of the *National*

Service Framework for Children, Young People and Maternity Services (Department of Health 2012) states:

> If you have to see the doctor or nurse or someone who can help because you are not so well – we want them to understand everything that you need to make you better. We also want them to ask you what YOU want, when YOU want it, and how YOU want it.

For young people, the style of delivery and language used is very different due to the recognition that young people are a defined group with their own needs, and their experiences should be used to develop and refine the services they use (Department of Health – Children and Young People 2011).

Bruner (1977) proposed that any subject could be taught to any child at any age provided the information was presented in a form the child could engage with. However, the acquisition of knowledge and/or skills can only be developed through the extension of previous experiences, which will develop as topics are repeatedly revisited as the child grows older (Bruner 1977).

Many children and young people hold naive and misleading concepts about bodily functions and their internal anatomy (Fleer and Leslie 1995) and these concepts are resistant to change, even into adulthood (Schmidt 2001). As a consequence, one of the key findings from Schmidt's research was the need to identify what the child or young person already knows about their body prior to providing new information.

In order to identify and 'challenge' misleading concepts that the child or young person may already have about their body and the way it functions, practitioners need to have sufficient body knowledge themselves and an awareness of how body knowledge is acquired by children and young people across the age range.

Fleer and Leslie (1995) proposed a five-step developmental sequence by which children develop an understanding of their bodies. The final stage was proposed for completion around the age of ten years.

FIVE-STEP DEVELOPMENTAL SEQUENCE FOR THE DEVELOPMENT OF BODILY AWARENESS

1. The internal organs are likely to be drawn inside and outside the child's body
2. A mixture of external items – such as facial features, decorative elements (bows and ribbons), and the navel – is likely to be included in the drawings of the internal body
3. The number of internal body parts drawn increases with age
4. The anatomical location of organs becomes more accurate with age
5. The connections between organs – at first partial and limited – become progressively more complete

(Fleer and Leslie 1995: 9)

Although no lower age limit was defined for when children can engage with information relating to the internal organs of the body, children between the ages of four and five years are believed to be the youngest age group that have the linguistic skills to participate in health-related issues (James 1995). However, early years practitioners have been encouraged since 2000 to promote discussions with pre-school children about 'the changes that happen to their bodies when they are active' by showing them that their hearts beat faster after exercise, and why this might be (Qualifications and Curriculum Authority 2000: 110). More recently it has been shown that children in the early years are able to engage with information about what lies inside their body (Tonkin 2007) and learning how the body works is now part of curriculum delivery within the early years (Early Education 2012). It has also been shown that children with chronic conditions may have an advanced knowledge about the internal organs related to their illness, but this is not always the case (Schmidt 2001).

Piaget proposed that in order for children to learn new concepts, they had to be at a certain stage of development (Pound 2005). Piaget believed that children under the age of seven were unable to think in the abstract and that children needed experience of real situations to think conceptually about what they cannot see (Bruce and Meggitt 2005). Although this reliance on stages has now largely been discredited, the importance of linking early experience to concept formation through concrete experiences remains (Bruce and Meggitt 2005). Pound (2005: 38), describing how Piaget's theories are put into practice, states 'learning is supported by action. Children need to experiment actively with materials and experience things in the real world to develop thought.' Gaudion (1997) suggests that this may help to explain why young children can identify internal features such as the heart and bones, which were the most commonly quoted internal body features during her research, due to sensory stimulation such as a beating heart or being able to feel bones, thereby providing an opportunity to relate abstract concepts to experience.

This may also explain why children under the age of nine were unable to link functioning of the lungs to inhalation and exhalation (Schmidt 2001). It is not obvious how the lungs work and although you can feel the rib cage expand and contract when breathing occurs, unless you have seen the lungs inflate and deflate as the rib cage moves, the link between form and function cannot be made. However, this provides a rationale for how anatomical and physiological information can be presented to children and young people in a way they can engage with, which links the application of knowledge to your practice.

Applied knowledge in practice

Knowledge of anatomy and physiology can provide explanations and rationales for the way in which investigations or treatment regimens are conducted (Schmidt 2001). Two examples of 'applied anatomical and physiological knowledge' are described below. These examples demonstrate how the provision of hands-on, practical experiences for children and young people may facilitate adherence to therapy or increased fluid intake to alleviate the effects of constipation through enhanced awareness of how the body functions.

Exploring the link between the 'press and breathe' technique in the management of asthma

Asthma affects the lungs, and in the United Kingdom over 1.1 million children have this chronic condition (NHS Choices 2012). Although asthma cannot be cured, it can be effectively managed, mostly by the inhalation of medication through an inhaler device. For the effective use of metered dose inhalers (MDIs), the patient needs to coordinate the activation of the device with breathing in at the same time (National Institute for Clinical Excellence 2000). For children aged 3–5 years of age, this is considered too difficult, so a spacer device is used with the inhaler which allows the medication to be inhaled over several breaths (National Institute for Clinical Excellence 2000). For children and young people aged 5–15 years of age, it is estimated that 50 per cent of 'press and breathe' MDI users are not optimizing delivery of the medication due to poor technique, due in part to poor coordination between activation of the MDI and inhalation (National Institute for Clinical Excellence 2002). This significantly reduces adherence to the therapy as spacer devices are then required, which may be inconvenient due to their portability and inducing feelings of stigma, which children may feel with their use (National Institute for Clinical Excellence 2002). Poor technique when using the inhaler can significantly reduce the amount of medication reaching the lungs, resulting in poor control of asthma (National Institute for Clinical Excellence 2002). This is a particular problem for younger children, where coordination of the 'press and breathe' MDI device does not occur.

When inhalation needs to be linked to an associated physical action, such as using an MDI; visualization and the provision of concrete experiences that children can relate to may enhance the compliance with instructions (Schmidt 2001; Gaudion 1997).

The breathing mechanism can be summarized as follows. When inhalation occurs, the diaphragm moves down, the external intercostal muscles pull the rib cage up and the lower part of the sternum moves forward. This expansion of the chest cavity causes a change in pressure, which makes the lungs inflate. Stretch receptors recognize when the lungs have expanded sufficiently, and instruct the lungs to deflate. At this point, the intercostal muscles and diaphragm relax, the diaphragm moves up, internal intercostals muscles depress the ribs and exhalation occurs.

Simple simulations of how the lung expands and contracts can be provided through blowing up a balloon and letting it deflate. If a more detailed explanation of the breathing mechanism is required, a model that simulates the breathing action can be made with the child or young person, or in advance as a display model. The chest is represented by a plastic bottle with the bottom removed. The other components are the trachea, bronchus, two main bronchi (single tube linked to two-way tubing) that go into the lungs (two balloons) and the diaphragm (balloon, with a tag to pull on, stretched across the bottom of the bottle). The model is a sealed system and pulling on the diaphragm simulates expansion of the chest cavity, the air pressure changes causing the balloons to inflate. When the diaphragm is released, the pressure returns to normal and the balloons deflate.

> Parker (1999) provides a step-by-step illustrated guide offering detailed instructions on how to build the model.
>
> An image for the completed model can be viewed via the following link from dkimages.com: www.dkimages.com/discover/home/health-and-beauty/human-body/Experiments/Oxygen-Supply/Oxygen-Supply-09.html.

Exploring the link between constipation and the functioning of the large intestine

Constipation is when you do not empty your bowels as often as you should and it is a relatively common childhood condition, affecting 5–30 per cent of the childhood population (National Institute for Health and Clinical Excellence 2010). One of the classic signs of constipation is pain when trying to pass stools (solid waste from the body), and this is often an important factor in constipation, which may create a vicious circle: 'the more it hurts, the more they [the child] hold back, the more constipated they get and the more it hurts' (NHS Choices 2013).

Activity 2.4

'It has been suggested that some healthcare professionals underestimate the impact of constipation on the child or young person and their family. This may contribute to the poor clinical outcomes often seen in children and young people with constipation' (National Institute for Health and Clinical Excellence 2010).

What are the signs and symptoms of constipation in children and young people and why might they cause social, psychological or educational consequences?

When the cause of constipation cannot be attributed to anatomical or physiological reasons following medical investigation and history taking, constipation is referred to as 'idiopathic'. Dietary interventions should not be used alone as the first line of treatment, but once the initial symptoms have been relieved through the use of laxatives, written information that promotes adequate fluid intake as part of a balanced diet should be provided. The way this information is presented depends on the child or young person's stage of development and includes, among other things, 'giving verbal information supported by (but not replaced by) written or website information in several formats about how the bowels work' (National Institute for Health and Clinical Excellence 2010: 28).

The main functions of the large intestine (also known as the large bowel) include the storage of solid waste products and the absorption of water from this toxic waste prior to its elimination as stools or faeces from the body. Waste material from the process of digestion enters the large intestine from the small intestine as a liquid. Excess water is absorbed as waste material passes through the large intestine, entering the descending colon as semi-solid waste. The longer this waste material remains in the large intestine, the more water is absorbed and the stools change in consistency as a result. Stool consistency is measured on the Bristol Stool Form Scale, which indicates intestinal transit time; children and young people with constipation are considered to pass stools identified as type 1: 'separate hard lumps, like nuts (hard to pass)' (National Institute for Health and Clinical Excellence 2010: 41).

As part of the multidisciplinary team, play specialists may be asked to assist in the management of idiopathic constipation, as this is often a long process that may take many months or years to rectify. Long-term care is often led by the Community Children's Nursing team, and techniques include sharing stories such as *Mr Poo: a children's story about constipation and stool withholding* (Cohn 2007). However, the following activity can be used to provide graphic visual simulation for children, young people and their carers of how constipation occurs as a result of extended intestinal transit time and why it is important to maintain adequate fluid intake as part of a balanced diet.

Activity 2.5

Try the 'Weetabix experiment'.
Weetabix represents waste material in the large intestine (plastic bag) and due to its high levels of absorbency it will soak up liquid that is added to it. The longer the Weetabix is left after the water has been added, the more water it absorbs, simulating how intestinal transit time affects stool consistency.

You will need three clear plastic sandwich bags, three small bowls or containers, a small cup, a jug of water, four Weetabix and a pair of scissors.

On each occasion, one Weetabix will be placed into a sandwich bag and crushed. One small cup of water is added and mixed with the Weetabix. When the appropriate time has passed, the top of the bag is gathered together and the contents are run into a corner of the bag. A hole is made in the corner at the bottom of the bag using the scissors and the contents are emptied into the small bowl. Before emptying the contents into the bowl, feel the consistency of the contents and when emptying the contents note the force needed to push the contents out of the bag.

Experiment 1 – leave the Weetabix and water in the bag for 30 seconds then release the contents into the bowl.

Experiment 2 – leave the Weetabix and water in the bag for three minutes then release the contents into the bowl.

Experiment 3 – leave the Weetabix and water in the bag for three minutes. Add a second Weetabix and mix together. Leave for a further minute then release the contents into the bowl.

Identify the stool type using the Bristol Stool Form Scale and identify how this experiment fits in with the theoretical considerations discussed earlier in the chapter.

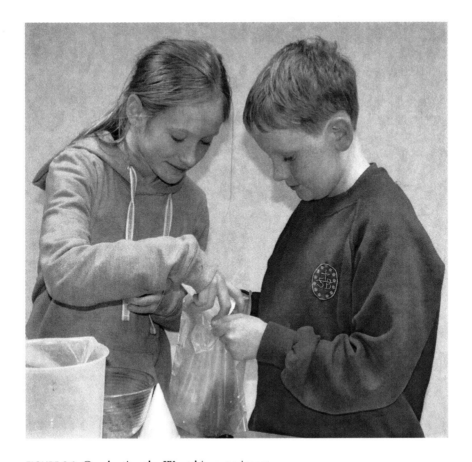

FIGURE 2.1 Conducting the Weetabix experiment.

Both of the examples given above identify the importance of how knowledge of anatomy and physiology can be applied in practice to provide concrete, hands-on practical experiences for children and young people. This promotes the linking of abstract concepts such as the functioning of the internal organs and body systems to treatment regimes in an effort to enhance compliance and promote active decision making by the child or young person.

Working with the multidisciplinary team

Applied knowledge may also be needed, as shown above, to enable you to fulfil your role within the multidisciplinary team (MDT). Nurses and allied health practitioners are required to learn about anatomy and physiology as part of their training and this knowledge is needed in order for their job role to be carried out effectively. For example, diagnostic and therapeutic radiographers use knowledge of surface anatomy that can be related to internal structures in both the imaging and treatment planning processes. The following provides one example of how strong professional links can increase the skills mix within the MDT, using applied anatomical and physiological knowledge to enhance the practitioner's contribution, enabling the sharing of appropriate information for the benefit of the child, young person and their family.

Although children and young people make up a high percentage of patients seen within imaging departments, they are not seen as a specialism, although specialist paediatric radiographers do exist (Society and College of Radiographers 2009). The value of the play specialist is recognized and they are seen as an integral member of the multidisciplinary team. Play specialists are expected to model techniques that other staff can adopt (Department of Health 2003) and managers must 'liaise with play specialists where appropriate to provide advice and/or services and education within the department' (Society and College of Radiographers 2009).

Play specialists are mostly used to prepare children and young people for advanced technological imaging procedures such as MRI, CT scanning and fluoroscopy, as well as routine procedures. This preparation includes 'explaining to a child what will happen' ... and visits to departments to enable patients to become familiar with equipment used for examinations' (Mathers et al. 2011: 22). Children and young people also require health-related information that helps inform the decision-making process (Mathers et al. 2011). Play specialists could also now assist in the preparation of child-friendly information that is tailored to the individual, using knowledge of child development and presentation formats. However, this requires an awareness of the imaging procedures involved and what part of the body or body system is being investigated. For example, 'Explain what an x-ray or scan is, i.e. a picture. Show them a real one of the appropriate body part – a non-scary one that shows clearly the bone you want to take the picture of. Build up a collection of old x-rays as part of your preparation box' (Tonkin et al. 2009: 21). That cannot be done without knowledge of the skeletal system, including the component bones and where they are situated.

Suggested answers to activities

Activity 2.1

Phlebitis – inflammation of a vein
Nephrolith – kidney stone
Gastroenteritis – inflammation of the lining of the membrane of the stomach and intestines
Meningioma – a slow-growing, encapsulated tumour arising from the meninges
Nephralgia – pain in the kidney
Bronchorrhoea – excessive discharge from the air passages of the lungs

Activity 2.2

Arthroplasty – the operative formation or restoration of a joint
Hysterectomy – surgical removal of the uterus
Orthodontics – a branch of dentistry dealing with irregularities of the teeth
Laparoscopy – visual examination of the inside of the abdomen by means of a laparoscope
Colostomy – surgical formation of an artificial anus by connecting the colon to an opening in the abdominal wall
Histology – minute structure of animal tissue as discernable with a microscope
Myotomy – incision of a muscle
Cardiology – the study of the heart and its actions and diseases
Nephrectomy – the surgical removal of a kidney
Cystogram – a radiographic image of the bladder
Neurology – branch of medicine concerned with the nervous system
Cystoscopy – the use of a cystoscope to examine the bladder
Arthroscopy – examination of a joint with an arthroscope

Useful sources of further information

Coeliac UK. A charity that provides advice and support for people with coeliac disease and dermatitis herpetiformis (DH): www.coeliac.org.uk.
Inner body: your guide to human anatomy online. Interactive learning tool that allows you to view all the main body systems and their component parts by scrolling over them: www.innerbody.com/htm/body.html.
Understanding medical words: a tutorial from the National Library of Medicine. This is an excellent website that guides you through medical terminology from a patient's perspective: www.nlm.nih.gov/medlineplus/medicalwords.html.
A–Z of medical conditions. Online listing of medical conditions with associated web links to reputable sources of information, support and guidance: www.dwp.gov.uk/publications/specialist-guides/medical-conditions/a-z-of-medical-conditions.

Further reading

Minnett, P., Wayne, D. and Rubenstein, D. (1998) *Human form and function*, London: Collins Educational.

References

Agenda for Change Project Team (2004) *The NHS Knowledge and Skills Framework. (NHS KSF) and the development review process*, London: Department of Health Publications.

Baines, P. (2008) Medical ethics for children: applying the four principles to paediatrics. *Journal of Medical Ethics*, 34(3): 141–145.

Bloom, B.S. (1956) *Taxonomy of educational objectives, handbook I: the cognitive domain*, New York: David McKay Co. Inc.

Bruce, T. and Meggitt, C. (2005) *Child care and education*, 3rd edn, Oxon: Hodder Arnold.

Bruner, J. (1977) *The process of education*, Cambridge, MA: Harvard University Press.

Cambridge Dictionary Online (2013a) *English definition of 'knowledge'*, Online. Available: http://dictionary.cambridge.org/dictionary/british/knowledge?q=knowledge (accessed 1 December 2013).

Cambridge Dictionary Online (2013b) English definition of '*condition*', Online. Available: http://dictionary.cambridge.org/dictionary/british/condition_1?q=condition (accessed 1 December 2013).

Chapman, A. (2009) *Bloom's taxonomy: learning domains*, Online. Available: www.business-balls.com/bloomstaxonomyoflearningdomains.htm (accessed 1 December 2013).

Cohn, A. (2007) *Constipation, withholding and your child: a family guide to soiling and wetting*, London: Jessica Kingsley Publishers Ltd.

CWDC (Children's Workforce Development Council) (2010) *The common core of skills and knowledge*, Leeds: Children's Workforce Development Council.

de Boo, M. (2001) The importance of science in early years education. Paper presented at The Education Show, Birmingham, March.

Department of Health (2003) *Getting the right start: National Service Framework for Children Standard for Hospital Services*, London: Department of Health.

Department of Health (2012) 2 is that we want to tell you the truth, Online. Available: http://webarchive.nationalarchives.gov.uk/+/www.dh.gov.uk/en/Publicationsandstatistics/Publications/PublicationsPolicyAndGuidance/Browsable/DH_4870695 (accessed 1 December 2013).

Department of Health – Children and Young People (2011) *You're welcome: quality criteria for young people friendly health services*, London: Department of Health.

Early Education (2012) *Development matters in the Early Years Foundation Stage (EYFS)*, London: Early Education.

Fleer, M. and Leslie, C. (1995) *What do I look like on the inside? Developing children's understanding about their bodies*, Watson, ACT: Australian Early Childhood Association.

Gaudion, C. (1997) Children's knowledge of their internal anatomy. *Paediatric Nursing*, 9(5): 7–14.

James, J. (1995) Children speak out about health. *Primary Health Care* 5: 8–12.

Jun Tai, N. (2008) *Play in hospital*, Online. Available: www.childrenwebmag.com/articles/play-articles/play-in-hospital (accessed 1 December 2013).

Mathers, S.A., Anderson, H. and McDonald, S. (2011) A survey of imaging services for children in England, Wales and Scotland. *Radiography*, 17: 20–27.

National Institute for Clinical Excellence (2000) *Guidance on the use of inhaler systems (devices) in children under the age of 5 years with chronic asthma: patient information*, London: National Institute for Clinical Excellence.

National Institute for Clinical Excellence (2002) *Inhaler devices for routine treatment of chronic asthma in older children (aged 5–15 years)*, London: National Institute for Clinical Excellence.

National Institute for Health and Clinical Excellence (2010) *Constipation in children and young people (CG99): diagnosis and management of idiopathic childhood constipation in primary and secondary care*, London: National Institute for Health and Clinical Excellence.

NHS Choices (2011) *NHS hospital services: children in hospital*, Online. Available: www.nhs.uk/nhsengland/aboutnhsservices/nhshospitals/pages/childreninhospital.aspx (accessed 1 December 2013).

NHS Choices (2012) *Asthma in children*, Online. Available: www.nhs.uk/conditions/asthma-in-children/pages/introduction.aspx (accessed 1 December 2013).

NHS Choices (2013) *Constipation and soiling in children*, Online. Available: www.nhs.uk/planners/birthtofive/pages/constipation.aspx (accessed 1 December 2013).

NHS Employers (2010) *Appraisals and KSF made simple: a practical guide*, London: NHS Employers.

Ofsted (2004) *Starting early: food and nutrition education of young children*, London: Ofsted Publications Centre.

Parker, S. (1999) *How the body works*, London: Dorland Kingsley Publishers Ltd.

Pound, L. (2005) *How children learn: From Montessori to Vygotsky – educational theories and approaches made easy*, Leamington Spa: Step Forward Publishing Ltd.

Qualifications and Curriculum Authority (2000) *Curriculum guidance for the foundation stage*, London: QCA Publications.

Rae-Dupree, J. and DuPree, P. (2007) *Anatomy and physiology workbook for dummies*, Hoboken, NJ: Wiley Publishing, Inc.

Schmidt, C. (2001) Development of children's body knowledge, using knowledge of the lungs as an exemplar. *Issues in Comprehensive Pediatric Nursing*, 24:177–191.

Society and College of Radiographers (2009) *Practice standards for the imaging of children and young people*, London: SCoR.

Tonkin, A. (2007) *Inside story*, Online. Available: www.nurseryworld.co.uk/nursery-world/news/1081492/inside-story (accessed 1 December 2013).

Tonkin, A., Mills, S. and Alexander, R. (2009) Let's play: part 2. *Synergy News*, December: 20–22.

3

THE CHILD, FAMILY AND SOCIETY

Vanessa Lovett

This chapter will provide an in-depth introduction to the child, family and society and allow you to reflect upon the practical application of theory when working with children and young people. 'Children' within the context of this chapter includes young people and they will not be referred to as a specific entity.

Chapter objectives

By the end of this chapter you should have an understanding of:

- the child, the family and society;
- significant theoretical perspectives and theories relating to the child's place in society and the influences of family and parenting style;
- the impact of societal influences and major research into the child's place within the family and in society;
- the different needs of children and families to support your work.

THE NHS KNOWLEDGE AND SKILLS FRAMEWORK

Communication

- maintains the highest standards of integrity when communicating with patients and the wider public

Equality and diversity

- interprets equality, diversity and rights in accordance with legislation, policies, procedures and good practice

(NHS Employers 2010)

THE COMMON CORE OF SKILLS AND KNOWLEDGE

Effective communication and engagement with children, young people and families

- Summarise situations in the appropriate way for the individual (taking into account factors such as background, age and personality)
- Recognise that different people have different interests in a situation and be able to work with them to reach the best and most fair conclusion for the child or young person

Child and young person development

- Understand that babies, children and young people see and experience the world in different ways
- Understand that families, parents and carers should be treated as partners and respected for their lead role and responsibility in addressing the specific needs of their child

(CWDC 2010)

Introduction

Every child is an individual, unique and shaped by their genetics and the environment, but what part do the family and society play in enabling a child to function and successfully navigate their way in the world? Children do not exist on the head of a pin; they are a part and a product of biology and experience. It is important for you to recognize that the children you work with within a healthcare setting come with predispositions and cultural experiences which may affect the way you work with them and their families.

This chapter will discuss different theoretical perspectives relating to the child's place in society. It will also consider the historical context of childhood and reflect on the impact that the family and parenting styles may have on the child's experience in society. It will also discuss the importance of socialization and the value that play and recreation have for enabling babies, children and young people to see and experience the world.

The child and childhood

Oxford Dictionaries (2013) define the child as 'a young human being below the age of puberty or below the legal age of majority', and England, Wales, Northern Ireland and Scotland agree that 'a child is anyone who has not yet reached their 18th birthday' (NSPCC 2013).

In the United Kingdom there is no single law that defines the age of a child. Article 1 of the United Nations Convention on the Rights of the Child, which was ratified by the UK government in 1991 (NSPCC 2013), states that a child 'means every human being below the age of eighteen years unless, under the law applicable to the child, majority is attained earlier'.

According to Giddens (1998: 36) 'Most of us tend to think of *childhood* as a clear and distinct stage of life. "Children" we suppose, are distinct from "babies" or "toddlers". Childhood intervenes between infancy and the onset of adolescence.' However, childhood is a fairly recent concept. It was only in the nineteenth century, with a growing awareness of the need for children's welfare, that a stage of childhood came to be recognized and valued. Prior to that, and in some countries today, children were viewed as small adults with roles and responsibilities to fulfil within the family. This might have included making a contribution to the family's economy through work, improving the family's social status through betrothal or undertaking responsibilities within the home. Pilcher and Wagg (1996) argue that childhood is a social construction which has been created to reflect the changing needs and values of society. This suggests that where children fit into society is not set but is different at different times and in different places. Therefore, we could say that despite the fact that humans go through the same stages of physical development, they are defined and constructed differently according to their culture. This can be taken further as childhood is not perceived in the same way by all societies. Some cultures do not necessarily see a difference between children and adults. An example of this is 'child soldiers', where their young age does not preclude them from fighting in wars, with the expectation that they can act like adults (Ansell 2005).

There are different sociological perspectives about childhood which reflect opposing views about whether childhood is a positive or a negative concept. For example, the New Right and Functionalists think that childhood is good because children need to be protected and they need a long process of socialization to understand the complexities of society, for example developing respect for authority. In this view, play and recreation are valuable vehicles for socialization. In contrast, Libertarians, Marxists and Feminists would suggest that it is expected that children make a contribution to the family as they see childhood as an artificial period of dependence and, even, a form of oppression. Play and recreation, therefore, are not valued. As part of this approach, it is not believed that children should be protected from some of the unpleasant realities of life such as death and violence.

Reflection

- Are the children you work with protected from the realities of their condition?
- How can play help children cope with the realities of their situation?

So what is childhood like in our contemporary society? What are children experiencing? We have laws to protect and safeguard children such as the Children Act 1989 and 2004, and children are provided with education opportunities until the age of 18. The United Nations Convention on the Rights of the Child (UNCRC) declares that 'the child, by reason of his physical and mental immaturity, needs special safeguards and care, including appropriate legal protection, before as well as after birth' (Office of the High Commissioner for Human Rights 2012). However, there is evidence that many children are not being protected (Laming 2009). The Bailey Review (2011), acting on parental concerns about how to protect their children from an inappropriate and increasingly sexualized culture, recommends that there is a clampdown on the sexualized 'wallpaper' surrounding children. Fisher and Gruescu (2011) suggest that services for children, such as maternity units, Children's Centres, play services and schools, can work to develop partnerships between family members and all those who wish to support children and young people.

In addition, many children in the United Kingdom are not achieving favourable educational outcomes compared with many other comparable countries, which has resulted in continuing government initiatives, most recently a revised National Curriculum (Department for Education 2013a) and new assessment framework (Department for Education 2013c). Work by the Department for Education has led to the following information:

> In maintained nursery, state-funded primary, state-funded secondary, special schools and pupil referral units, 18.3 per cent of pupils were known to be eligible for and claiming free school meals, compared to 18.2 per cent in 2012.

The Department for Education produces statistics relating to schools, pupils and their characteristics and it showed that the

> average size of key stage 1 classes taught by one teacher on the census day in January 2013 was 27.3, compared to 27.2 in January 2012. The number of key stage 1 classes reported as having more than 30 pupils on the census day, lawfully and unlawfully, was 2,299 (from a total of 56,597 classes), 4.1 per cent of all key stage 1 classes, up from 2.7 per cent in January 2012.
>
> *(Department for Education 2013b)*

Research undertaken by Cassen and Kingdon (2007) at the London School of Economics, based on work by the Joseph Rowntree Foundation, suggests that

> eligibility for free school meals is strongly associated with low achievement, but significantly more so for White British pupils than for other ethnic groups. Other indicators of disadvantage, such as the neighbourhood unemployment rate, the percentage of single-parent households and the proportion of

parents with low educational qualifications, all measured in the immediate area round the student's home, are also statistically associated with low achievement.

This is the experience of some of the children who you will be supporting in your healthcare setting.

Reflection

- Are these children stakeholders in society?
- Article 12 in the UNCRC (Office of the High Commissioner for Human Rights 2012) says that children's views should be taken seriously, but is that always possible?
- How would you be able to ensure this in a healthcare setting?

McLeod (2008) describes the work of Bee (1992), explaining that in order for a child to function within the family and society they need to be able to develop a sense of themselves and their identity. McLeod suggests that the sense of being separate and different from others is the most fundamental aspect of the 'self-scheme' or self-concept, which leads to child's developing perception of the self as a constant. The child comes to understand that they exist as a separate being from others and that this existence will continue over time and space. Lewis (1990) suggests that this 'awareness of the existential self' might start from when the baby is as young as two to three months and is initiated, partly, because of how the child interacts with the environment. Examples of this interaction are the social smile or where the child pushes a tower of bricks and it falls over. Lewis (1990) goes on to describe that the child, when they have come to understand that they exist as a separate entity that has their own experiences, becomes conscious that they are an object in the world as much as any other. They realize that they can be experienced as an object, which has its own properties. Children begin to classify these properties of the 'self' including size, age, gender and skill. Early self-classifications are gender ('I am a girl') and age ('I am 3'). You may be familiar with small children's inclination to be very precise about their exact age.

Rogers (1959) in Taylor (2012) suggests that self-concept is made up of three different parts:

1. how you see yourself – self-image;
2. the value you have for yourself – self-esteem or self-worth;
3. what you wish you were really like – ideal self.

Children's experiences combined with their temperaments will affect these components.

Kuhn's (1960) exploration of self-attitude identified five main groups. These were:

1   social groups and classifications
2   ideological beliefs
3   interests
4   ambitions
5   self-evaluations.

Which categories did your self-description fall into?

Schubert (1998) explains that Cooley in 1918, believed that it is a human predisposition to be social in nature, and that much information about the world is derived from interaction with others, including the idea of the 'self'. Cooley is most well-known for the concept of the 'looking glass self', which is the idea of how people appear to others. He saw this as an essential piece of the development of self-image. Cooley developed this further, suggesting that human society functions 'organically' and can only be healthy and effective if individuals consider the needs of others and are not restricted by the primacy of their own needs. We can see here that there is an argument for the nature side of debate and, indeed, Pinker (2003) would argue that the primacy of family ties and predisposition to share are innate. This would indicate that the child is born with the facility and drive to belong to a social group and that first social group is usually the family.

The family

In 1949 Murdock looked at 250 societies and suggested that there was evidence that a 'type of family' existed in those examined. His definition of a family as a social group included:

> Common residence; economic co-operation; reproduction; adults of both sexes, two of whom maintain a socially approved sexual relationship; one or more children (own or adopted) of these adults.
>
> *(Holborn et al. 2009)*

Murdock's definition suggests a nuclear family structure. The Free Dictionary (2013) defines the nuclear family as 'A family unit consisting of a mother and father and their children.' The nuclear family, as a family structure, is a fairly recent creation of Western society. It could be seen as being less efficient than an extended family model, with its benefits including child rearing and care, as well as the care of older family members. However, Murdock did identify that the nuclear family is widespread, either as an independent unit or as the core unit within an extended family (Holborn *et al.* 2009). However, what constitutes a family has changed considerably since Murdock's time and a definition can be a tricky subject. Beck and Beck-Gernsheim (1995) state:

> It is no longer possible to pronounce in some binding way what family, marriage, parenthood, sexuality or love mean, what they should or could be; rather these vary in substance, norms and morality from individual to individual and from relationship to relationship.

The changing nature of the family structure is reflected in current data from the Office for National Statistics (2013), which suggest the number of children being born to unmarried couples will increase to over 50 per cent by 2016.

You will be working with children from a variety of families and it is important to be aware of the impact that they have on each individual child. You could consider the family to be a micro-level society in which the roles, responsibilities, status and hierarchy of wider society are reflected. Bronfenbrenner developed the ecological systems theory in 1979 to explain how factors within the child and in the child's environment influences how that child grows and develops (Pound 2009). He proposed that the environment is made up of different features or levels which impact on children's development. These include the 'microsystem', the 'mesosystem', the 'exosystem' and the 'macrosystem'. The microsystem is the narrow, immediate environment in which the child lives. The microsystems children have will include close relationships or organizations they interact with, such as family or caregivers, nursery or school. The interactions between these groups or organizations will have an impact on the way the child grows (Pound 2009). There is a correlation between the extent of these relationships and places and the extent to which the child will be able to grow and develop. Additionally, there is mutuality between how a child acts or reacts to these people in the microsystem and how they treat the child in return. The child's temperament, based on individual genetic and biologically influenced personality traits, influences how others treat them (Oswalt 2008). The child's temperament is also related to 'goodness of fit', described in 1977 by Thomas and Chess as the compatibility between environment and a child's temperament (Zentner and Bates 2008). Goodness of fit facilitates the achievement of potential – for example, when adults meet children's individual learning styles (Culpepper 2008). Cowles and Aldridge (1992) suggest that poorness of fit can also happen if the child's temperament is not valued and accommodated, and Zentner and Bates 2008 note that 'adequacy (i.e. fit) of parental responses to this temperament' is equally important.

It is in this context that the child first experiences their culture, and the norms and values that are important; socialization is the process through which this takes place. Watson suggested that it is through adults shaping the behaviour of children that children learn what is required to fit in with their culture (Shaffer 2005). However, this suggests a behaviourist emphasis and does not consider the impact of nature. Pinker (2004) considers the balance of nature versus nurture and states:

> At this point it is tempting to conclude that people are shaped both by genes and by family upbringing: how their parents treated them and what kind of home they grew up in. But the conclusion is unwarranted. Behavioral genetics allows one to distinguish two very different ways in which people's environments might affect them. The shared environment is what impinges on a person and his or her siblings alike: their parents, home life, and neighborhood. The unique environment is everything else: anything that happens to a person that does not necessarily happen to that person's siblings.
>
> *(Pinker 2004: 10)*

Bowlby (1958) proposed that babies are predisposed to form attachments with their primary caregiver which suggests that human biology leads us to be social beings. Santer *et al.* (2007) suggests that when children have a strong, secure relationship with their immediate carers, play exchanges develop spontaneously. Implicit in this is that because time and attention is given to the child, they gain a sense of worth.

Reflection

- How much time and attention are you able to give to individual children when you play with them?
- Have you seen that children develop a sense of worth from your interactions?

As the child develops through the process of maturation and experience, peers become significantly more important to them. This is part of their development of self-identity and children seek out others for a variety of reasons, such as to reinforce aspects of their identity or to try to change their own self-image. Fisher and Gruescu (2011) identify that, in 2007, Unicef placed the UK at the bottom of the league of developed countries in relation to children's overall wellbeing and, in particular, in relation to children's experience of family and friends. It found that neglect of children has not reduced over the years and child poverty has become constant and is now more likely to worsen because of the weaker economic environment. Both of these factors significantly inhibit children's ability to form the friendships and networks that enable them to progress in the world.

Reflection

• What opportunities are you able to provide for young people to socialize in their recreational activities?

In 2013 Unicef United Kingdom published *Report card 11* and the United Kingdom was placed sixteenth out of 29 countries in the new Unicef table of child wellbeing. Although this showed an improvement and 86 per cent life satisfaction reported by UK children, the report noted that improvements were not consistent across all areas and there was much work to be done (Unicef United Kingdom 2013).

In 1980 Erikson, building on the work of Sigmund Freud, proposed stages of psycho-social development; each one to be successfully achieved through conflict resolution in order to progress to the next. The early stages are to do with relationships within the family. However, during the latency stage (approximately 6–12 years) external influences become increasingly important (Nevid 2008). In this latent or school-age stage, the teacher and school become increasingly important in influencing self-identity. Erikson argued that if the child did not develop an industrious approach, progression from this stage would not be possible and the child could be plagued with feelings of inferiority or incompetence for the long term (Kincheloe and Horn 2007). It is also during this stage that peers become increasingly important.

> The discovery of the limits of family influence is not just a debunking exercise, but opens up important new questions. The finding that much of the variance in personality, intelligence, and behaviour comes neither from the genes nor from the family environment raises the question of where it does come from. Judith Rich Harris has argued that the phenomena known as socialization – acquiring the skills and values needed to thrive in a given culture – take place in the peer group rather than the family.
>
> *(Pinker 2004: 11)*

Another finding from Unicef Innocenti Research Centre (2007) said that British children had the 'worst relationships on average in the developed world'. Only about one-third of 'British families said they ate together regularly. Britain was also ranked last when relationships among 11–15 year olds were examined.'

We have recently seen an increasing trend for children and young people to become part of gang culture. Some children and young people are turning to peer role models within their community for a sense of belonging and self-identity rather than to their families. An example of this is described in an article about girls who are becoming members of gangs:

> Gang-involved girls navigate harmful environments and relationships. According to the study from the Centre for Mental Health, young women who had 'histories of parental imprisonment, poor parental mental health, parental substance misuse, or neglect' were three to five times more likely to be gang-involved than other girls who were screened. In addition, they were three times more likely to be identified as victims of sexual abuse and four times more likely to have been excluded from school.
>
> *(Firmin 2013)*

There is some indication here, then, that parents can have an impact on children and young people's life choices. Parental life choices may cause them to be unable to meet the needs of their own children. Although we cannot attribute gang membership to parenting styles, at this point it is worth considering the impact that parenting styles can have on children and young people. Cherry's (2013) discussion on the effects of parenting styles on children's developmental outcomes is relevant here. She says that, in addition to Baumrind's initial 1991 study of 100 pre-school children, the studies which other researchers have undertaken lead to significant conclusions about the impact of parenting styles on children.

- 'Authoritarian parenting styles generally lead to children who are obedient and proficient, but they rank lower in happiness, social competence and self-esteem
- Authoritative parenting styles tend to result in children who are happy, capable and successful' (Maccoby 1992)
- 'Permissive parenting often results in children who rank low in happiness and self-regulation. These children are more likely to experience problems with authority and tend to perform poorly in school
- Uninvolved parenting styles rank lowest across all life domains. These children tend to lack self-control, have low self-esteem and are less competent than their peers' (Cherry 2013)

Reflection

- Which parenting style may be the most likely to lead to children joining gangs?
- What is your experience of the impact of parents on their children in your care?
- How do you work with parents whose parenting style you don't agree with?

Chan and Koo (2011: 396) agree with Cherry, and go further, saying:

> It is parenting style that matters. Specifically, authoritative parenting is associated with higher self-esteem and subjective well-being, and lower odds of smoking, getting involved in fights, or having friends who use drugs. As regards educational outcomes, where class origin and parental education are significant predictors, parenting style also has significant net associations. When compared with authoritarian or permissive parenting, authoritative parenting is associated with better GCSE results and higher odds of staying on in education beyond school-leaving age. Parenting style is an additional, rather than a mediating, factor of educational attainment, and given that there is no net association between parenting style and social class, one could say that parenting style is statistically independent to class.

This provides further demonstration of the complexity of childhood and family life (Flatters 2012). Peterson and Green (2009) cite Epstein *et al.* (1993) in stating 'family roles are patterns of behavior by which individuals fulfill family functions and needs'. There is not scope within this chapter to look at all family roles, but a contemporary issue of significance is the role of fathers.

Rosenburg and Wilcox (2006) describe the work of Popenoe (1996), who was at the forefront of research into the new field of study about fatherhood. It was noted that fathers were more than 'just "second adults" in the home, and that fathers who were involved brought many positive benefits to their children "that no other person is as likely to bring"'. This has particular resonance as the Centre for Social Justice (CSJ) has identified that 'more than a million children in the UK are growing up without a father, according to a report on family breakdown' (Marshall 2013). The CSJ claimed the number of lone-parent families increases by 20,000 a year and 'will reach more than two million by the next General Election in 2015. Some of the poorest areas of the United Kingdom are becoming "men deserts" because there are so few visible male role models for children' (Marshall 2013).

The Institute for the Study of Civil Society (2013) explains that previously, psychologists who studied the development of children focused, almost without exception, on the relationships children had with their mothers. Now, their position has changed and there is recognition that fathers have a specific and crucial role in the nurture and guidance of children. Experts such as Pruett (1987) have been advocating that fathers can be as nurturing and sensitive with their babies as mothers. This influence continues as their children grow and fathers assume additional roles such as guiding their children's intellectual and social development. It is also important to note that even when a father is 'just playing' with his children, he is nurturing their development.

Barth and Parke (1993) say that there are further beneficial outcomes when fathers are involved during their child's school years, such as helping their children to adjust during those difficult first years of school. They suggest that supportive fathers have children with fewer problems, such as excessive absence or poor exam results at school. King and Sobolewski (2006) contribute to this discussion and have found that even limited attention, warmth and affection from fathers, even with periods of absence, means their children benefit from their influence. This may be in relation to adapting to new experiences, emotional stability and the ability of how to relate to others. You may have observed the impact that fathers have on helping their children to adjust to the new experience of being in a healthcare setting.

Reflection

- In what ways do you think children benefit from fathers' involvement in the healthcare setting?
- Do children have the opportunity to explore gender role models in their play in the healthcare setting? What would the benefit of this be for children?

Although we have not considered all roles within the family, it is possible to identify further roles within the family structure; father, mother, siblings and members of the extended family. Each of these carries status and, within each family, there is a hierarchy. This may depend on culture, personality and temperament, or even financial contribution. Nevertheless, it is this hierarchy and sense of status that is the child's first experience of the fact that each of us has our own place within a social framework. When looked at more widely, hierarchy and status are fundamental concepts to understand in order to navigate wider society.

Society

Cambridge Dictionaries Online (2013) describe society as:

> A large group of people who live together in an organized way, making decisions about how to do things and sharing the work that needs to be done. All the people in a country, or in several similar countries, can be referred to as a society.

The level of decision making depends on the role and level of responsibility, but this definition highlights the importance of working together. What has taken place in the family and through children's early social experiences will set the template for how they expect society to function. If the child has had negative experiences of others because of discrimination, prejudice or abuse, the impact on their self-image and sense of self will have been significant and will influence how they engage with society. On the other hand, if a child has had nurturing relationships and positive experiences they will have a more hopeful view of what society has to offer.

So, society is made up of individuals and groups. If we focus on the individual's experience of society, some interesting considerations in relation to the physical body emerge. Kennedy and Kennedy (2010) cite Douglas (1970: 93), who stated:

> ... the social body constrains the way the physical body is perceived. The physical experience of the body ... sustains a particular view of society. There is a continual exchange of meaning between the two kinds of bodily experience so that each reinforces the other.

From this they infer that control over the body exerts social control over both the individual and groups of people. Everyday expressions such as 'spineless' or thick-skinned' bring together the body with symbolic meaning to express moral sentiments.

Kennedy and Kennedy (2010) go further in suggesting that body parts may also be used as social metaphors to convey moral statements about how people act or should act. Indeed, the implication can be applied to the shape and weight of our bodies in relation to whether we conform to social norms or societal values. The following commentary provides a good overview of how society can work together with the help of the government to address major health concerns.

As we have seen, self-image and identity are significant in influencing how and why a child becomes part of a wider social group. One significant contemporary issue is that of childhood obesity and GOV.UK (2013a) states that 30 per cent of children aged between two and 15 years of age are overweight or obese. One of the causes of this may be the increasing sedentary habits of children and young people due to the increasing availability and use of technology, particularly within the home (Public Health England 2013).

GOV.UK (2013b) says that only one-third of boys and a quarter of girls meet the recommendation for at least 60 minutes of physical activity per day and the statistics 'show that nearly 30 per cent of adults are active for less than 30 minutes per week'. The Department of Health has introduced the 'Get active to get healthy' initiative, together with 'more than £5 million of funding to encourage children and families to exercise more' (GOV.UK 2013b). One of the most interesting initiatives involves an attempt to revive street play. Play England will be allocated a budget of £1.1 million to:

> ... help residents and encourage children and families to play together on their streets, reviving old favourites like hopscotch and hide-and-seek. This funding will enable Play England help residents close their roads from time to time to allow children and families to play out in a safer environment.
>
> *(GOV.UK 2013b)*

This is an interesting development as a recent survey undertaken by Play England (2013) showed that only 23 per cent of children play outside on a weekly basis, with 28 per cent of adults citing intolerant neighbours as a key factor in their reluctance to allow their children to play outdoors. Clearly, society will need to decide on how to react to this latest contentious issue.

Reflection

- Are you able to provide opportunities for exercise and outdoor play for children in your setting?
- What are the limitations for these in a healthcare setting?

This chapter has considered sociological perspectives, contemporary issues and government attempts to address rapidly changing circumstances in society. The children and families who you will be working with are subject to these issues and circumstances, and it is important for you to develop a reflective approach as to how and why children and their families function as they do, so that you can provide appropriate support.

References

Ansell, N. (2005). *Children, youth and development*, Oxon: Routledge.

Bailey, R. (2011) *Letting children be children*, Norwich: The Stationery Office.

Barth, J.M. and Parke, R.D. (1993) Parent–child relationship influences on children's transition to school. *Merrill-Palmer Quarterly*, 39: 173–195.

Beck, U. and Beck-Gernsheim, E. (1995) *The normal chaos of love*, Cambridge: Polity Press.

Bowlby, J. (1958) The nature of the child's tie to his mother. *International Journal of Psycho-Analysis*, 39: 350–373.

Cambridge Dictionaries Online (2013) *English definition of 'Society'*. Online. Available: http://dictionary.cambridge.org/dictionary/british/society_1?q=society (accessed 14 December 2013).

Cassen, R. and Kingdon, G. (2007) *Tackling low educational achievement*. Online. Available: http://eprints.lse.ac.uk/43735/1/Tackling%20low%20educational%20achievement(lsero).pdf (accessed 14 December 2013).

Chan, T.W. and Koo, A. (2011) Parenting style and youth outcomes in the UK. *European Sociological Review*, 27(3): 385–399.

Cherry, K. (2013) *Parenting styles: the four styles of parenting*, Online. Available: http://psychology.about.com/od/developmentalpsychology/a/parenting-style.htm (accessed 14 December 2013).

Cowles, M. and Aldridge, J. (1992) *Activity-oriented classrooms*, Washington, DC: National Education Association.

Culpepper, S. (2008) *The temperament trap: recognizing and accommodating children's personalities*, Online. Available: www.earlychildhoodnews.com/earlychildhood/article_view.aspx?ArticleID=673 (accessed 14 December 2013).

CWDC (Children's Workforce Development Council) (2010) *The common core of skills and knowledge*, Leeds: Children's Workforce Development Council.

Department for Education (2013a) *2014 National Curriculum*. Online. Available: www.education.gov.uk/schools/teachingandlearning/curriculum/nationalcurriculum2014 (accessed 14 December 2013).

Department for Education (2013b) *Statistical first release: schools, pupils and their characteristics, January 2013*. Online. Available: www.gov.uk/government/uploads/system/uploads/attachment_data/file/207670/Main_text-_SFR21_2013.pdf (accessed 14 December 2013).

Department for Education (2013c) *Assessing without levels*. Online. Available: www.education.gov.uk/schools/teachingandlearning/curriculum/nationalcurriculum2014/a00225864/assessing-without-levels (accessed 14 December 2013).

Firmin, C. (2013) We must identify girls at risk from gangs, *Guardian*, 21 May.

Fisher, D. and Gruescu, S. (2011) *Children and the Big Society: backing communities to keep the next generation safe and happy*, Online. Available: www.actionforchildren.org.uk/media/810373/children_and_the_big_society.pdf. (accessed 14 December 2013).

Flatters, P. (2012) *Viewpoint: children have never had it so good*. Online. Available: www.bbc.co.uk/news/magazine-16409882 (accessed 14 December 2013).

Free Dictionary (2013) *Nuclear family*. Online Available: www.thefreedictionary.com/nuclear+family (accessed 14 December 2013).

Giddens, A. (1998) *Sociology*, Oxford: Blackwell.

GOV.UK (2013a) *Reducing obesity and improving diet*. Online. Available: www.gov.uk/government/policies/reducing-obesity-and-improving-diet (accessed 14 December 2013).

GOV.UK (2013b) *Press release: get active to get healthy*. Online. Available: www.gov.uk/government/news/get-active-to-get-healthy (accessed 14 December 2013).

Holborn, M., Langley, P. and Burrage, P. (2009) *Haralambos and Holborn: sociology themes and perspectives student handbook: AS and A2 level*, 7th edn, London: Harper Collins.

Institute for the Study of Civil Society (2013) *How do fathers fit in*. Online. Available: www.civitas.org.uk/hwu/fathers.php (accessed 14 December 2013).

Kennedy, P. and Kennedy, C.A. (2010) *Using theory to explore health, medicine and society*, Bristol: The Polity Press.

Kincheloe, J.L. and Horn, R.A. (eds) (2007) *The Praeger Handbook of education and psychology, Volume 1*, Westport, CT: Praeger Publishers.

King, V. and Sobolewski, J. (2006) Non-resident fathers' contributions to adolescent well-being. *Journal of Marriage and the Family*, 68(3): 537–557.

Kuhn, M. (1960) Self-attitudes by age, sex, and professional training. *The Sociological Quarterly*, 1(1): 39–54.

Laming, Lord (2009) *The Protection of Children in England: A Progress Report*, London: The Stationery Office.

Lewis, M. (1990) Self-knowledge and social development in early life. In: Pervin, L. (ed.), *Handbook of personality: theory and research*, New York: Guilford Press.

Maccoby, E.E. (1992) The role of parents in the socialization of children: an historical overview. *Developmental Psychology*, 28: 1006–1017.

McLeod, S. (2008) *Self concept*. Online. Available: www.simplypsychology.org/self-concept.html (accessed 14 December 2013).

Marshall, P. (2013) One million kids 'without dads'. *ITV News*. 10 June 2013. Online. Available: www.itv.com/news/story/2013-06-10/one-million-uk-children-grow-up-without-a-father (accessed 24 March 2014).

Nevid, J.S. (2008) *Psychology concepts and applications*, 3rd edn, Boston, MA: Houghton Mifflin Company.

NHS Employers (2010) *Appraisals and KSF made simple: a practical guide*, London: NHS Employers.

NSPCC (2013) *Legal definition of a child*. Online. Available: www.nspcc.org.uk/Inform/research/questions/definition_of_a_child_wda59396.html (accessed 14 December 2013).

Office for National Statistics (2013) *Births in England and Wales, 2012*. Online. Available: www.ons.gov.uk/ons/dcp171778_317196.pdf (accessed 14 December 2013).

Office of the High Commissioner for Human Rights (2012) *Convention on the Rights of the Child*. Online. Available: www.ohchr.org/en/professionalinterest/pages/crc.aspx (accessed 14 December 2013).

Oswalt, K. (2008) *Urie Bronfenbrenner and Child Development*. Online. Available: www.mentalhelp.net/poc/view_doc.php?type=doc&id=7930 (accessed 14 December 2013).

Oxford Dictionaries (2013) *Definition of child in English*. Online. Available: http://oxforddictionaries.com/definition/english/child (accessed 14 December 2013).

Peterson, R. and Green, S. (2009) *Families first: keys to successful family functioning – family roles*. Online. Available: http://pubs.ext.vt.edu/350/350-093/350-093.html (accessed 14 December 2013).

Pilcher, J. and Wagg, S. (eds) (1996) *Thatcher's children? Politics, childhood and society in the 1980s and 1990s*, Oxon: Routledge Falmer.

Pinker, S. (2003) *The Blank Slate: The Modern Denial of Human Nature*, London: Penguin.

Pinker, S. (2004) *Why nature & nurture?* Online. Available: http://pinker.wjh.harvard.edu/articles/papers/nature_nurture.pdf (accessed 14 December 2013).

Play England (2013) *Unwelcoming communities stop children playing out*. Online. Available: www.playengland.org.uk/news/2013/08/unwelcoming-communities-stop-children-playing-out.aspx (accessed 14 December 2013).

Pound, L. (2009) *How children learn 3: contemporary thinking and theorists*, London: Practical Pre-School Books.

Pruett, K. (1987) *The nurturing father*, New York: Warner Books.

Public Health England (2013) *How healthy behaviour supports children's wellbeing*, London: Public Health England.

Rosenburg, J. and Wilcox, W.B. (2006) *The importance of fathers in the healthy development of children*. Online. Available: www.childwelfare.gov/pubs/usermanuals/fatherhood/chaptertwo.cfm (accessed 14 December 2013).

Santer, J., Griffiths, C. and Goodall, D. (2007) *Free play in early childhood: a literature review*, London: Play England.

Schubert, H.J. (ed.) (1998) *Charles Horton Cooley on self and social organization*, Chicago, IL: University of Chicago Press.

Shaffer, H.R. (2005) *Social development*, Oxford: Blackwell Publishers.

Taylor, C. (2012) *Empathic care for children with disorganized attachments: a model for mentalizing, attachment and trauma-informed care*, London: Jessica Kingsley Publishers.

Unicef Innocenti Research Centre (2007) *Child poverty in perspective: an overview of child well-being in rich countries*, Florence: UNICEF Innocenti Research Centre.

Unicef United Kingdom (2013) *Report card 11: child well-being in rich countries – a comparative overview*, Florence: Unicef UK.

Zentner, M. and Bates, J.E. (2008) Child temperament: an integrative review of concepts, research programs, and measures. *European Journal of Developmental Science*, 2(1/2): 7–37.

4

CHILD DEVELOPMENT IN PRACTICE

Vanessa Lovett, Claire Weldon and Alison Tonkin

This chapter will demonstrate how knowledge of child development can be applied in practice, particularly with regard to observing and assessing the developmental stage of children and young people. When the assessment process is done effectively, it enables planning (covered in Chapter 5) to be undertaken, to provide developmentally appropriate play and recreation resources and activities within the setting.

Chapter objectives

By the end of this chapter you should have an understanding of:

- why having and using knowledge about the development of children and young people is important and how it can be used within your practice;
- how to assess the development of children and young people through the 'observation, assessment and planning cycle';
- how to evaluate and update your own knowledge of theoretical perspectives of development and the implications of these for your practice.

THE NHS KNOWLEDGE AND SKILLS FRAMEWORK

Communication

- Shares and engages thinking with others
    - Accurate information given
    - Appropriate information given

Personal and people development

- Takes responsibility for meeting own development needs
    - People feel they have the knowledge and skills to do their jobs
    - People feel responsible for developing their own expertise

(NHS Employers 2010)

THE COMMON CORE OF SKILLS AND KNOWLEDGE

Effective communication and engagement with children, young people and families

- Summarise situations in the appropriate way for the individual (taking into account factors such as background, age and personality)
- Present genuine choices to children and young people, explaining what has happened or will happen next and what they are consenting to
- Recognise that different people have different interests in a situation and be able to work with them to reach the best and most fair conclusion for the child or young person
- Know when and how to refer to sources of information, advice or support from different agencies or professionals in children's or adult services

Child and young person development

- Encourage children or young people to value their personal experiences and knowledge
- Know how to interact with children and young people in ways that support the development of their ability to think, learn, and become independent
- Know that development includes emotional, physical, sexual, intellectual, social, moral and character growth, and that these can all affect one another
- Understand that play and recreation that is directed by babies, children and young people – rather than by adults – has a major role in helping them to understand themselves and the world. It also helps them to build confidence and realise their potential.

(CWDC 2010)

Introduction

All children and young people are different. The study of child development is essential in enabling practitioners to work effectively with children and young people to provide for their individual care, learning and developmental needs. The Cambridge Dictionary Online (2013) describes development as 'when someone or something grows or changes and becomes more advanced'. Children's development should not be thought of as progressing in a linear way. Children do not, for example, just develop physically while they are learning to sit, crawl and walk. They are encountering new social experiences, gaining confidence and self-reliance and developing ways to communicate with others. In this sense, we can think of development as a holistic process. In this way you can see how areas of development are linked and overlap and the child's development can be seen as a complex and interwoven web. Recognition of the child as an 'integrated being' is important and practitioners need to be aware that 'the development of each area of functioning is dependent on other areas' (Meisels and Atkins-Burnett 2000: 232). This can be demonstrated through a relatively simple task, such as a child naming a picture. According to Meisels and Atkins-Burnett (2000) this requires language acquisition, sensory, motor and cognitive skills, as well as the emotional capabilities to relate to others. They conclude by stating 'to consider only one area of development in isolation from the others leaves unrecognised the influence of the other areas and may obscure our understanding of the child's abilities and challenges' (Meisels and Atkins-Burnett 2000: 232).

Practitioners could encounter children and young people at different stages of their development, and being in a healthcare setting can have an effect on how the child's development progresses or regresses. It is, therefore, essential that you are able to assess children's stage of development and identify factors influencing that development, to ensure that you reflect on the holistic development of the whole child (Lindon 2010). To do this you will need to develop skills of observation in order to make accurate assessments of the stage of development reached, the child's individual needs and how to plan to meet those needs. In order to make accurate and valid assessments it will be important for you to refer to valid sources of information against which to measure developmental progress. Much work and research has been put into developing a set of developmental milestones that practitioners can refer to, which will be considered later in the chapter. It will be important for you to use these and not refer to some of the less well researched websites that populate the internet. It will also be important for you to be aware of your own ideas, views and assumptions that you might hold about the children and young people you work with. We have all been subject to influences which have contributed to our ideas about how children should or should not be, and it is all too easy to let these influence our assessments. However, as a professional practitioner it is very important that you do not allow any preconceptions to influence your assessment, which should be sound, accurate and based on evidence. It is only when you have clear observational findings linked to developmental milestones that you can evaluate what stage the child or young person has reached, what they need and what you need to provide to meet those needs.

This chapter will explore different methods of observation, valid sources for developmental milestones, evaluation skills and how to apply these in your role as a practitioner. It will also enable you to reflect on different theoretical perspectives and consider how these can influence your practice.

Why is knowledge of child development important?

Practitioners' knowledge of child development across the healthcare sector has been raised as an issue, particularly for those who do not routinely work with children and young people on a regular basis (Kennedy 2010). Kennedy suggests that training for practitioners needs to:

... address not only matters specific to the care and welfare of children and young people, but matters such as how to work in teams, how to see the child or young person holistically [and] understanding of the development of children and young people.

(Kennedy 2010: 13)

However, this is not just a problem for those working within the NHS or the health sector. Brandon *et al.* (2011) point out that child development training across differing professional sectors is patchy and lacks consistency. Brandon *et al.* (2011) reviewed a small sample of serious case reviews, focusing on child and family practitioners' understanding of child development. They concluded that:

Overall it would appear that there is scope for improvement in child development training for all professionals working with children. A good in-depth knowledge of normal development is essential if practitioners are to grasp the nuanced understanding that meeting developmental milestones is not a sufficient guide to good development or to safety.

(Brandon et al. 2011: 21)

So how can knowledge of child development enhance your professional practice and what benefits can this bring to the children, young people and families you work with?

Without knowledge of child development, you may not know what the expected developmental levels should be. Within a healthcare setting, a lack of awareness may result in asking a child to perform a task that is too difficult or belittles them, and this could reduce the chances of a successful procedure or investigation (Tonkin and Weldon 2013). Therefore, developing this knowledge will enable you to identify needs and possible concerns and be confident in sharing your findings with the multidisciplinary team.

Opportunities for children to demonstrate some aspects of development may be more limited in the context of a hospital environment, where development may also regress. For example, a child may refuse to feed themselves or may start wetting themselves when they had previously been dry. It is therefore important not to rely on one occasion of observation and to recognize factors which might be affecting the child's stage of development. It is also worth noting that 'the same environment may have different effects on children who are born with different characteristics' (Boyd and Bee 2012: 8).

Reflection

Have you noticed that children's behaviour has been affected by their:

- illness?
- healthcare environment?

Did you do anything as a result?

When discussing development it is very important to consider the debate about 'nature versus nurture'. Some aspects of development may be influenced by genetic factors (nature), while environmental factors (nurture) may play a significant role in influencing development (Boyd and Bee 2012). It is generally agreed that both factors can affect children's development both positively and negatively.

How to assess the development of children and young people through observation

The process of assessing a child's level of development follows a sequence that should start with the family, as they will generally be able to provide useful information that can give a background context for the child. If the child or young person is old enough, they can be active and willing participants in the assessment process. Data can be collected through a variety of methods over a period of time, and collated and evaluated to clearly identify the developmental stage the child is at, resulting in the creation of 'plans of action' that will help the child to move forward (Meisels and Atkins-Burnett 2000).

Observation is defined as 'the action or process of closely observing or monitoring something or someone ... the ability to notice things, especially significant details ... a statement based on something one has seen, heard, or noticed' (Oxford Dictionaries 2013a). Observation is a key part of the planning cycle, as shown in Figure 4.1, and the information gained through the observation is the starting point of a cyclical process. In order to carry out an observation to identify how the child

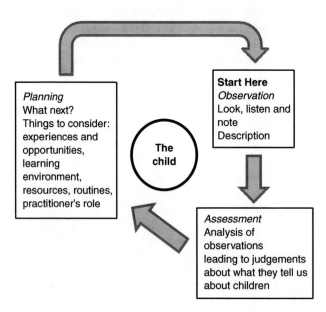

FIGURE 4.1 The observation, assessment and planning cycle (source: adapted from Department for Children, Schools and Families 2007).

or young person is developing you will need to be attentive, accurate, objective and unbiased. The more detailed your observation, the more 'raw data' you will have to evaluate the developmental level. This will enable you to make a valid assessment of the child which will help to plan for their needs and enables you to 'understand and consider the child's current interests, development and learning' (Department for Children Schools and Families 2007: 1).

Observation techniques

There are many observation techniques and it can be useful to think of them as part of an 'observation toolkit'. Siren Films (2010: 2) state that 'as well as learning observation skills it is also important to be able to identify which type of observation is required'. Each observation technique provides a certain type of information and you select the observation technique from your 'toolbox' depending on what you want to find out. This means it is important that you have a clear aim and focus before you start to observe so that 'useful conclusions can be drawn' (Siren Films 2010) when the raw observational data is analysed. All techniques have advantages and disadvantages and you will find that different techniques are useful in different contexts. Table 4.1 summarizes the main observational techniques and suggests possible considerations when choosing or using each technique.

Narrative observations are good for providing a very detailed account of what the child is doing, but to maintain the level of concentration and detail is difficult. Therefore a narrative observation is usually undertaken over a relatively short period of time, such as 5–10 minutes. A shorter and much more concise narrative observation can be recorded on a post-it note and this type of technique is good for sharing observations as part of a key person system. However, this system will only work if the information from post-it notes is collated and this can be time consuming (Tassoni 2008).

Taking photographs or images without consent within NHS settings can result in serious professional misconduct and therefore when considering whether to take pictures within the healthcare setting, ensure permission is given from the appropriate person before doing so. It is worth checking to see if the setting has a policy relating to visual and audio recording, even if you are not including patients within your recordings. For example, Tameside Hospital Foundation NHS Trust (2012) has a policy covering 'photography, video/DVD recording and filming' that specifically relates to patients and staff and this comprehensive policy provides clarity in terms of what is permissible and the scope of what is covered.

Tassoni (2008) suggests that recording methods should be practical and user-friendly, not just for those doing the observation, but also those who will use the recorded data, which may include parents. The 'Target Child' or TC method was devised in the 1970s by the Oxford Pre-school Research Project to study concentration (Hobart *et al.* 2004). This method records what the child is doing and any language used through narrative documentation, as well as the social context and activities that the child is engaged in through the use of pre-coded letters and

TABLE 4.1 Overview of observation techniques and things to consider

Technique	Activity	Things to consider
Written record or narrative accounts	This is a detailed written account that records what the child is doing, including all interactions and language used	How long would a typical narrative observation take?
Video and photographs	Static (photographs) and dynamic (video) images that provide a visual record of what the child is doing	What restrictions are there to using video recordings or photographs within a healthcare setting?
Target child	This specialized technique typically takes place over a ten-minute period with ten one-minute blocks to record everything that occurs under specified headings using predetermined coding	Do you think you need training to be able to use the predetermined codes and template to be able to use this method effectively?
Checklists and tick charts	Need to prepare the observation template in advance depending on what you are 'checking', e.g. achievement of developmental milestones – these are 'ticked off' when they have been seen	If a child does not demonstrate competency of the milestone when you observe them, does this mean they are not competent?
Time sample	Using a preprepared table, the child is observed at regular intervals, e.g. every 15 minutes, to record what they are doing at that particular moment in time	How practical is this type of observation for one person to undertake over a sustained period of time e.g. a whole morning?
Event sample	Using a preprepared table, each time a specified behaviour occurs it is recorded and the background context is documented	Would you let the child or young person being observed know that you are monitoring their behaviour?
Tracking	This is used to track the movements of the child within the setting. It requires a floor plan that shows the set-up of the equipment and activities, allowing the child's movements to be tracked	How could you document the amount of time spent at each activity or piece of equipment? Why might this be useful?
Post-it notes	Post-it notes can be used to record very brief, spontaneous observations to demonstrate specific examples of behaviour or achievement	How might these observations help other members of the team who also care for the child?

symbols. For trained observers this provides a very detailed observation, but the interpretation also requires knowledge of what the coding stands for and it can be difficult to summarize the observation data in a precise manner (Hobart *et al.* 2004).

Tick charts can be useful for providing an overview of how children are progressing but they should not be used on their own as they provide a 'snapshot' of what the child can achieve. It should be noted that competency for a particular task or developmental milestone should not rely solely on tick charts and checklists, but these should be used in conjunction with other observations. Tassoni (2008) suggests adding comments to tick charts can be beneficial and this enables additional evidence to be linked to the recorded information. This also applies to tracking observations, which record the movements of a child over the course of a given period of time. The longer they last, the more complicated they become, especially if the child frequently moves between activities. Although adding the time spent at each activity may provide additional information, it can also make the observation more muddled and difficult to interpret.

When there are concerns over particular aspects of behaviour, sampling observations can be used that record when predetermined criteria are met. For example, time sampling will use predetermined times to observe what is happening at the allotted time slot. This is usually done at regular periods over a sustained period of time, e.g. every 15 minutes or every hour over the course of a morning or the whole day. This can be useful for providing an overview of what a child does over the course of a day or can be used to identify the frequency of a particular aspect of behaviour (Siren Films 2010). This can be undertaken by 'whoever is free' at the time to do the observation, so can be done as a team, as long as someone has responsibility for ensuring the observations are done at the required time slot and there is consistency in terms of the depth and detail that needs to be recorded. Alternatively, event sampling focuses on a particular event or behaviour and, as such, the length or frequency of observation is dependent on when and for how long the behaviour occurs. Being aware that you are being observed can alter how people behave and, therefore, gaining consent to undertake observations that focus on particular aspects of behaviour can be difficult, especially as children get older and are aware of the implications of any observations that you may undertake.

Activity 4.1

If you have the opportunity to work with a colleague, undertake a double observation of the same activity or child and compare notes on completion.

- Did you gather similar information and focus on the same aspects?
- Was the depth and detail within each of your observations similar?
- If the content of your observations varied, why do you think this may be?

Prior to undertaking observations, you may need to seek permission from parents and be conscious about the importance of maintaining confidentiality. It is good practice for parents to have access to their child's observations; the child or young person may also see it, so consider the language and terms used when writing your observation. It is also worthwhile considering the impact that observation can have on the child or young person you are observing. The child or young person's behaviour may alter for a variety of reasons, such as feeling self-conscious, uncooperative or 'playing to the gallery'. Therefore, it is important that you plan your observations to make the process as unobtrusive as possible.

For all observations it is important to write the date and time of when it was carried out. This can help you to identify whether the child's behaviour is different at different times of day or if there are changes over a period of time. It is also helpful to provide a brief overview of what was happening just before the observation took place, including details such as where the observation took place and who was around, particularly if an adult was present. The child's age in months and years as well as their date of birth and gender should also be recorded.

Assessment of the observation

Once you have carried out the observation, the processes of assessment and evaluation can begin. The more depth and detail the observational raw data provides, the more detailed the assessment can be.

For assessment purposes, child development is generally divided into five main areas: physical development (including fine and gross motor skills); intellectual (or cognitive) development; language development; emotional development; and social development, which may also include spiritual development (PILES). In order to make an accurate assessment, start by referring to developmental milestones which will give an indication of how the child or young person is developing. A milestone can be described as 'a significant stage or event in the development of something' (Oxford Dictionaries 2013b), and this demonstrates that milestones can show us key points in the process of development. Not all children reach milestones at the same age for a variety of reasons. Nevertheless, they are useful indicators of how development is progressing and help to identify strategies that can be put in place to move the child forward.

It is important to use valid and reliable developmental charts and a list of some appropriate sources of developmental milestones has been provided under 'useful sources of information' at the end of the chapter.

Using all of the observational raw data and linking it to the range of developmental milestones associated with PILES provides a rich source of evidence that extends beyond the original aim. It also ensures consideration of the interdependency of functions and helps bring the assessment back to the holistic child.

The needs of children change as they grow and have new experiences. This is particularly evident in adolescence as hormonal changes impact on the young person's body and emotions. This may have a significant impact on the body image of the young person which may, in turn, affect their self-image and sense of identity. The social and emotional needs of a young person are different from those of the younger child, and peers become increasingly important during the teenage years. This is considered in more detail in Chapter 3.

Having defined 'where the child is at' the final stage of the planning cycle can now be undertaken. Strategies to improve the experience for children and young people in healthcare settings, the compilation of play plans and the provision of a range of play and recreational activities can be designed to meet the identified developmental needs of the child.

How to evaluate and update your own knowledge of theoretical perspectives of development and the implications for your practice

A theory is a principle or idea that is proposed, researched and generally accepted as an explanation (Herr 2012). Developmental theories provide insights into how children grow, learn and engage with the world in which they live. Knowledge about theory becomes useful when it is specifically linked to practice. Tables 4.2–4.3 were designed to show how specific age and developmental factors may cause difficulties for children and young people when undergoing diagnostic imaging procedures and how these may be overcome within practice. Theories are helpful for understanding and guiding developmental processes. Theories can be useful decision-making tools (Herr 2012). Another reason to learn about theory is that it provides a complementary framework to the knowledge of developmental milestones. That is, theory gives us reasons or evidence that allow us to explain and predict how children may react when certain factors come into play. Table 4.2 (age range of 0–10 years) and Table 4.3 (age range of 11–18 years) demonstrate how the imaging of children and young people within a diagnostic imaging department may be affected by different factors at different stages of their lives. This information can be used as a guide and linked to other aspects of healthcare.

The next section looks at six theorists whose theories are often used to explain what is happening in certain situations. They can also help to provide ideas to consider or things you can do to enhance the experience that children, young people and their families have when using the services you offer.

The following summaries and associated tables were originally developed for the e-Learning for Healthcare online module *Image interpretation of the paediatric skeleton: child development – relevance to imaging children* (Tonkin and Weldon 2013). The module was written to promote knowledge about child development for diagnostic radiographers, linking developmental theory to practice to enhance the imaging experience. This is particularly important for children who may have long-term conditions requiring regular attendance to a healthcare setting over a sustained period of time.

Table 4.4 provides an overview of the six featured theorists. Following is a more detailed description of each theory.

TABLE 4.2 Factors to consider when imaging children in the age range 0–10 years

Factors	Age range (years)	Factors for consideration	Solutions
Separation from carers Being alone	0–2	Has difficulty expressing anxiety Reluctance to be held or touched by an unfamiliar person Senses parental stress	Ask parents/carers to do as much as possible before and during the procedure, e.g. positioning child Prepare area in advance Explain procedure to parent/child
	2–5	Difficulty expressing anxiety	Explain to child where parent/carer will be if they cannot stay Prepare area in advance
Pain	0–2	Has difficulty localizing pain Reluctance for an area which hurts to be touched/moved	Check pain relief is sufficient; wait if not Adapt procedure if necessary
	2–5	Can give a basic history and can usually localize area of pain	Discuss symptoms to establish relationship
Overstimulation	2–5	Can be unsettled by unfamiliar sounds/people/equipment Difficulty following multiple instructions	Reduce number of people involved/in the room Reduce noise Use familiar items: dummy, comfort toys/blanket
	5–10	Difficulty processing lots of information	Use short sentences Don't give too many instructions in one go
Change in routine	0–2	Has difficulty if needs/routine are not met	Be aware of feeding/sleep times and the result of disrupting them
Fears, expectations and previous experiences	2–5	Fear of pain during procedure Fear of the dark Fear of the unknown Difficulty understanding explanation of procedure as it is an abstract concept	Show pictures/preparation books prior to procedure Discuss previous experiences Clarify understanding/experiences from parent/carer
Communication	0–10	Understands single words in context Uses single words Understands simple sentences Asks questions Uses simple sentences Follows directions Follows others' body language Responds to simple instructions Re-tells details of a simple past event in the correct order Can express knowledge and understanding and ask appropriate questions	Speak clearly and use actions to support instructions Use a running commentary Show photographs and stories of procedure Give clear directions Give children 'thinking time' Use statements rather than questions Give possible answers to questions Give the child the opportunity to ask questions

Source: Weldon and Weldon (2012a).

TABLE 4.3 Factors to consider when imaging children in the age range 11–18 years

Factors	Age range (years)	Considerations	Solutions
Waiting times	11–18	Poorly managed waiting times can lead to increased anxiety and irritability	Reduce waiting times if possible
		Long waiting times can lead to disruptive behaviour	Display current waiting time
			Recommend bringing an activity to booked appointments
Compliance		Fear of procedure	Check understanding of procedure
		Misconceptions originating from peers, internet or social media	Explain procedure
			Send information/factsheets with appointment
Modesty		Modesty can be a more important issue for young people than a procedure itself	Allow child to change in cubicle away from parents/others
		Self-conscious about wearing hospital clothing	Respect privacy
		Cultural factors – gender, religious	Recommend bringing suitable clothing from home. Include in information/factsheet
		Age of puberty varies	
Consent		Understanding of procedure and implications	Clarify and document understanding
		Consider and present contraindications and interactions of procedure	Discuss consent issues with young person
			Establish Gillick competence if applicable
		Inconsistency in understanding between young person and parent/carer over planned treatment	Explain how procedure is in their best interest and supports the long-term treatment process
Understanding	11–18	Age and stage of understanding may be different	Encourage questions
		May not want to admit to not understanding	Check understanding of procedure and document if necessary
			Send information/factsheets with appointment

Source: Weldon and Weldon (2012b).

TABLE 4.4 Summary of theorists, their theory and how this may be reflected through practice

Theorist	Theory	Link to practice
Albert Bandura	Social learning theory	Role modelling and engagement. Interaction between thinking, the environment and behaviour affects how children and young people react to situations they are in
Jerome Bruner	Stage model of development Spiral curriculum	Representation of experience changes over time, which will define how you engage with, and present information to, children and young people
Erik Erikson	Eight stages of psycho-social development that run across the lifespan	How children and young people engage and communicate with you is dependent upon the stage they have 'mastered'
Susan Isaacs	With gentle support and encouragement, children and young people can work out how the world works for themselves	Positive praise and gentle encouragement works better than harsh words and criticism Children and young people learn through practical, hands-on tasks with functioning tools
Jean Piaget	Sequential stage theory for children's cognitive development	Awareness of the differing stages may help to identify the level and type of information children and young people can engage with
Burrhus Skinner	Operant conditioning	Use of positive reinforcement (stickers and certificates)

Albert Bandura (1925–present)

Bandura's best known theory is social learning theory. This has many sub-elements within it; just three of these are covered in Table 4.5.

Jerome Bruner (1915–present)

Bruner is a developmental psychologist who has focused on the construction of knowledge with particular reference to the cultural aspects of learning. Bruner's work emphasizes that children are always learning and that through the use of a spiral curriculum, any subject can be taught at any stage of a child's development, provided it is taught in a way the child can engage with. Bruner developed a three-stage model that sought to explain how children's representation of experiences is changed into knowledge in a loosely sequential manner. Movement between the stages is negotiable and depends on the child's level of experience (Pound 2005) (Table 4.6).

TABLE 4.5 Three elements from Bandura's social learning theory

Reciprocal determinism	*Self-efficacy*	*Role-modelling*
Our thinking, behaviour and the environment are constantly interacting and changing the way we think and feel. This means that what, how and where we do things are linked together and each will affect the other (Allen and Gordon 2011).	This is at the centre of Bandura's theory and describes how an individual personally perceives and responds to differing situations. It links observational learning, social experience and reciprocal determination to define the individual's own beliefs as to how well they can manage and succeed on any given task (Allen and Gordon 2011).	Most human behaviour is learned through observation, which can lead to imitation. The stages leading to imitation are attention (see it), retention (remember it), reproduction (use it) and motivation (have reason to use it) (Allen and Gordon 2011).
Considerations	*Considerations*	*Considerations*
An unfamiliar environment may adversely affect behaviour. This can be minimized through small changes to the environment. The influence of the differing factors change according to the age/developmental stage of the child/young person.	Knowing that the amount of effort someone will put into a task depends on whether or not they think the outcome will be successful. This means alternative strategies may be required to help a child who has previously had an unsuccessful investigation because they did not follow the required preparation. It is important for young people to be able to contribute to their own healthcare planning.	When engaging with young people, the way you interact with them will affect the way they interact with you. You may be able to encourage a child or young person to remain still during a procedure or intervention by promoting the use of imitation and role modelling.

TABLE 4.6 Bruner's three-stage 'modes of representation' model

Enactive mode (0–1 years)	Iconic mode (1–6 years)	Symbolic mode (7+ years)	Link to practice
Involves physical action. Knowledge is stored mainly through action or movement, which cannot necessarily be described through pictures or words (Pound 2005).	Knowledge is stored mainly through visual images and pictures (Pound 2005).	Experience is represented through a range of symbolic systems such as numbers, words or other types of coding systems (Pound 2005).	Bruner's work can be used in a variety of ways to prepare children and young people for investigations and procedures. It may be useful to have diagrams or pictures to accompany verbal information

This use of a spiral curriculum 'approach' can fit into the provision of information for children and young people across the differing age ranges and the variation in iconic and symbolic representation across the differing developmental ages and stages is often reflected within 'children and young people' areas of hospital websites (as discussed in Chapter 10).

Erik Erikson (1902–1994)

Erikson proposed that there are eight stages of psycho-social development that run across the lifespan. Although he did not identify how development occurred, each stage is defined by a 'central dilemma or crisis' (Pound 2005) that has to be confronted and 'mastered' successfully to enable progression onto the next level. However, 'crises' that are not successfully mastered will not prevent movement through the stages but may cause problems in the future (Table 4.7).

Susan Isaacs (1885–1948)

Isaacs believed that children, with gentle support and guidance, could determine how the world works for themselves. Isaacs emphasized the emotional needs of children and taught that 'adults should never be sarcastic towards children, or break promises made to them ... and their questions should be answered seriously and respectfully' (Pound 2005). Isaacs was hugely influential in the late 1920s and 1930s and her legacy includes the use of naturalistic observations that focus on children in their natural environment as opposed to assessing them within contrived test situations.

Activity 4.2

Look at the following features of Isaacs' work: how could these apply in practice?

- 'Quiet, positive encouragement, showing the child what to do and how to do it is far more effective than scolding or punishment, or emphasis on what he should not do. Successes should be emphasized; failures should be minimized; and above all any feelings of shame or of hostility should be avoided' (Isaacs, cited in Pound 2005)
- Isaacs, influenced by the work of Montessori, provided functioning tools and working equipment that could perform the task they were intended for. This enabled children to engage in exploration and encouraged their curiosity through hands-on, practical experiences that were embedded in the real world.

The Kennedy Review suggests that 'a lack of training in treating children and young people may lead staff to treat them inappropriately, however unintentionally' (Kennedy 2010: 31).

TABLE 4.7 The first five stages of Erikson's psycho-social development theory linked to practice

Stage	Description (taken from Pound 2005)	Application in practice
Trust vs mistrust (birth to 1 year)	'The first task is to develop a sense of trust or comfort in their caregivers, environment and self'	Consistent care is important and parental involvement should be encouraged to meet both social and physical needs
Autonomy vs shame and doubt (1–3 years)	'Young children are learning to exercise independence … the child needs to be supported in making choices and decisions'	Encourage exploration of the environment and materials through the use of play. Exposure to appropriate language is important
Initiative vs guilt (3–6 years)	'The young child's developing desire to master the environment'	Assess understanding and provide age-appropriate explanations; increase opportunities for control
Industry vs inferiority (6 years to adolescence)	'Children are keen to master intellectual and social challenges but failures may lead to feelings of inferiority and incompetence'	Provide structured opportunities for preparation, using peer interaction where possible; more emphasis on 'being involved'
Identity vs identity diffusion (12–20 years)	'Young people need to explore their own identity – failure to do so may lead to confusion'	Privacy is very important, as are relationships; where possible, promote control, choice, independence and self-expression

Isaacs' comments above clearly identify that adults need to treat children and young people with respect and honesty. The *You're Welcome quality criteria: making health services young people friendly* publication (Department of Health – Children and Young People 2011) attempts to address this by giving clear guidance on how staff should provide appropriate services (Tonkin and Weldon 2013).

Jean Piaget (1896–1980)

Piaget believed that children are active learners who use firsthand experience and prior experiences to enable them to learn. Children imitate people and their experiences and transform these into symbolic behaviour. Piaget developed a sequential stage theory and believed the child had to fully master one stage before they could progress onto the next. However, Piaget underestimated children and young people's capabilities through the testing procedures that were used, but his theory provides a useful overview of how children develop their thinking characteristics, if the age bands are treated with a degree of caution (Pound 2005) (Table 4.8).

Burrhus Frederic Skinner (1904–1990)

Skinner is one of the best-known behaviourist theorists. Skinner believed that all behaviour is learned and therefore can be shaped. Skinner emphasized the positive

TABLE 4.8 Piaget's stage theory of cognitive development and possible implications for practice

Stage of development	Characteristics (Pound 2005)	Implications
Sensori-motor (0–2 years)	Learning is developed through physical action and the child's senses	Environment is key … factors such as noise and touch
Pre-operational (2–7 years)	Objects are represented by words, supporting play with ideas Logic rests on incomplete ideas	Lack of abstract thinking means explanations need concrete examples (Figure 4.2). Feelings cannot be controlled by reason
Concrete operations (7–12 years)	Logical thought emerges and experiences are categorized	Enjoy explanations but these need to be tangible or seen
Formal operations (12+)	Manipulation of abstract ideas and a systematic approach to solving problems	Capable of reasoned discussion and see implications. Avoid displaying vulnerability. Reasoning may depend on their mood

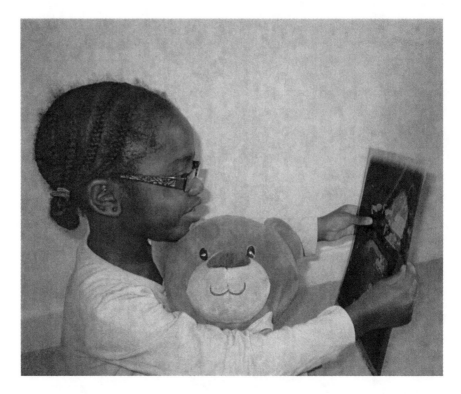

FIGURE 4.2 Children require explanations using concrete examples.

nature of rewards, believing negative reinforcement to be counter-productive. Table 4.9 shows two elements of Skinner's work, what this could mean for you as a practitioner and how these elements link to other theories.

This chapter has covered the topic of child development and identified how the developmental level of a child or young person can be assessed through the observation process. Once this has been established, the next stage of the process is to plan age- and stage-appropriate play and recreational resources and activities for children and young people. This is covered in Chapter 5.

Useful sources of additional information

Boyd, D. and Bee, H. (2012) *The developing child*, 13th edn, Oxford: Pearson.

Christie, D. and Viner, R. (2005) Adolescent development. In: Viner, R. (ed.), *The ABC of Adolescence*, Oxford: Wiley-Blackwell: 1–4.

Meggitt, C. (2012) *Child development: an illustrated guide* 3rd edn, Oxford: Pearson Education.

Sheridan, M. (2001) *From birth to five years: children's developmental progress*, London: Routledge.

Sheridan, M., Sharma, A. and Cockerill, H. (2014) *From birth to five years: children's developmental progress*, 4th edn, Oxon: Routledge.

TABLE 4.9 Two elements of Skinner's behaviourist theory and how they link to practice and other theories

Operant conditioning	Breaking things down	Links to other
Building on the work done by Pavlov in relation to classical conditioning, Skinner identified how the use of reinforcement could further modify behaviour.	Skinner identified that children could perform complex tasks that had previously been thought too complicated, if the task was broken down into smaller tasks, with each task being positively reinforced as it was learned (Pound 2005).	The link to social learning theory has raised awareness of the need to:
If you want to encourage the behaviour, a positive stimulus is provided. If you want to discourage the behaviour, a negative stimulus is provided (Pound 2005).		• manage behaviour – both in terms of encouraging desired behaviour and conflict resolution
		• increase awareness of how observed behaviour is repeated through positive and negative reinforcement (Pound 2005).
Considerations:	*Considerations:*	*Considerations:*
When a child has successfully completed a procedure, you can offer a reward (usually in the form of a sticker or certificate). The 'Beads of Courage' programme uses the concept of positive reinforcement to 'reward' successful completion of investigations, procedures or treatment.	Breaking information down into 'bite-sized chunks' when preparing children to undergo a complex procedure may help them to turn the procedure into a manageable task.	Children (and young people) enjoy receiving 'rewards' and these can be used by way of role modelling to other children undergoing similar procedures. This may also allow the sharing of experiences in a positive and supportive manner.

References

Allen, S. and Gordon, P. (2011) *How children learn 4: thinking on special educational needs and inclusion*, London: Practical Pre-School Books.

Boyd, D. and Bee, H. (2012) *The developing child*, 13th edn, Oxford: Pearson.

Brandon, M., Sidebotham, P., Ellis, C., Bailey, S. and Belderson, P. (2011) *Child and family practitioners' understanding of child development: lessons learnt from a small sample of serious case reviews*, London: Department for Education.

Cambridge Dictionaries Online (2013) *English definition of 'development'*. Online. Available: http://dictionary.cambridge.org/dictionary/british/development_1?q=development (accessed 3 December 2013).

CWDC (Children's Workforce Development Council) (2010) *The common core of skills and knowledge*, Leeds: Children's Workforce Development Council.

Department for Children, Schools and Families (2007) *Effective practice: observation, assessment and planning*, Nottingham: DCSF Publications.

Department of Health – Children and Young People (2011) *You're welcome: quality criteria for young people friendly health services*. London: Department of Health.

Herr, J. (2012) *Working with young children*, 7th edn, Tinley Park, IL: Goodheart-Wilcox Publisher.

Hobart, C., Frankel, J. and Walker, M. (2004) *A practical guide to child observation and assessment*, 3rd edn, Cheltenham: Nelson Thornes.

Kennedy, I. (2010) *Getting it right for children and young people: overcoming cultural barriers in the NHS so as to meet their needs*, London: Department of Health.

Lindon, J. (2010) *Understanding child development: linking theory and practice*, 2nd edn, London: Hodder Education.

Meisels, S.J. and Atkins-Burnett, S. (2000) The elements of early childhood assessment. In Shonkoff, J.P. and Meisels, S.J. (eds), *Handbook of early childhood intervention*. New York: Cambridge University Press.

NHS Employers (2010) *Appraisals and KSF made simple: a practical guide*, London: NHS Employers.

Oxford Dictionaries (2013a) *Definition of 'observation' in English*. Online. Available: www.oxforddictionaries.com/definition/english/observation?q=observation (accessed 3 December 2013).

Oxford Dictionaries (2013b) *Definition of 'milestone' in English*. Online. Available: www.oxforddictionaries.com/definition/english/milestone?q=milestone (accessed 3 December 2013).

Pound, L. (2005) *How children learn: from Montessori to Vygotsky – educational theories and approaches made easy*, Leamington Spa: Step Forward Publishing Ltd.

Siren Films (2010) *Child observation no. 7: time & event sampling – user notes*. Online. Available: www.sirenfilms.co.uk/store/usernotes/1235660055.580LID0.pdf (accessed 3 December 2013).

Tameside Hospital Foundation NHS Trust (2012) *Visual and audio recordings of patients policy (photography, video/DVD recording and filming) Version 2*. Online. Available: www.tamesidehospital.nhs.uk/documents/photographypolicy.pdf (accessed 3 December 2013).

Tassoni, P. (2008) *Penny Tassoni's practical EYFS handbook*, Harlow: Heinemann.

Tonkin, A. and Weldon, C. (2013) *Image interpretation of the paediatric skeleton: child development – relevance to imaging children (602-0605)*, HEE e-Learning for Healthcare.

Weldon, C. and Weldon, J. (2012a) The theory behind imaging children, *Synergy News*, September.

Weldon, C. and Weldon, J. (2012b) The theory behind imaging young people, *Synergy News*, October.

5

PLAY AND RECREATION

Claire Weldon and Helen Peck

This chapter will discuss the importance of play and recreation in healthcare settings. It will look at theoretical approaches and the role of healthcare professionals in implementing play and recreation. The benefits of play will be discussed, as well as strategies to improve the experience for children and young people in a healthcare setting through writing play plans and providing a range of play and recreational activities.

Chapter objectives

By the end of this chapter you will be able to:

- identify the theoretical perspectives that underpin the role of play in healthcare settings;
- identify the benefits of play in healthcare settings;
- develop and write play plans;
- work with a range of professionals within the multi-professional team to promote the role of play and recreation.

THE NHS KNOWLEDGE AND SKILLS FRAMEWORK

Communication

- Identifies the impact of contextual factors on communication
- Adapts communication to take account of others' culture, background and preferred way of communicating
- Develops partnerships and actively maintains them

Health safety and security

- Works in a way that complies with legislation and trust policies and procedures on health, safety and risk management

(NHS Employers 2010)

THE COMMON CORE OF SKILLS AND KNOWLEDGE

Effective communication and engagement with children, young people and families

- Use clear language to communicate with all children, young people, families and carers, including people who find communication difficult, or are at risk of exclusion or under-achievement
- Be able to adapt styles of communication to the needs and abilities of children and young people who do not communicate verbally, or communicate in different ways
- Present genuine choices to children and young people, explaining what has happened or will happen next and what they are consenting to
- Be aware of different ways of communicating, including technological methods. Understand barriers to communication, which could include poverty, cultural or faith requirements, disability, disadvantage or anxiety about accessing services.

Child and young person development

- Understand that play and recreation that is directed by babies, children and young people – rather than by adults – has a major role in helping them to understand themselves and the world. It also helps them to build confidence and realise their potential.
- Know how to use theory and experience to reflect upon, think about and improve practice. Know how to take responsibility for meeting your professional development needs.

(CWDC 2010)

Introduction

The role of play in a hospital environment can help to provide a normalizing experience for children and young people, can help to speed up recovery time and provide a method to express fear and reduce stress and anxiety (Jun-Tai 2005). For children that are long-term patients or are hospitalized for a long period of time, play can assist with a child's development and reduce regression. Play can also help children and young people to understand treatments, prepare them for medical procedures and offer ways of coping, using a range of specialized play techniques. Play is considered so important to the holistic needs of children that the United Nations Convention on the Rights of the Child deems play to be a fundamental right and, according to Article 31, 'all children have the right to play and relaxation, which should include a wide range of recreational activities, including those reflecting culture' (Unicef, 2013). This will be discussed in more detail later in the chapter.

It is not easy to define the terms 'play' and 'recreation'. Play usually describes the activities that children engage in. Play activities are usually freely chosen and support the emotional development of children. Children can play alone or with others and it is usually an enjoyable experience. Play in a healthcare context involves 'normal' play that enables children to play with familiar objects, together with more specialized techniques such as play preparation, post-procedural play and distraction therapy (Lindon 2002). Recreation often refers to activities and pastimes that are enjoyable, such as hobbies and sports that young people and adults participate in. In a healthcare setting these should be provided in an age and stage appropriate environment. Most playrooms cater to the needs of young children so the provision of a teenage room and a more 'grown up' looking space is particularly important for this age group, who need books, magazines and health information appropriate to them, and a range of up-to-date resources to support their needs (Department of Health – Children and Young People 2011).

This very practical chapter will begin by exploring theoretical perspectives surrounding the provision of play and recreation activities and resources, paying particular attention to the role of the environment. It will then go on to describe how health issues or illness can affect the opportunities to engage in play and adaptations that may be needed. Finally, this chapter looks at the role of the multidisciplinary team and how play and recreation can enhance service provision for children and young people.

Theoretical perspectives

Understanding theory is important because theoretical perspectives offer differing perspectives. Developmental theory, which was discussed in Chapter 4, showed how most children and young people develop through a recognizable pattern of development. This allows services to respond to the needs of children and young people in a developmentally appropriate manner (Kennedy 2010). Theory can also help to enhance the service offered in unexpected ways. For example, being aware of how to manage the environment will help to minimize stress-related anxiety, which may cause variations in behaviour that are hard to manage. The following brief overview of three play-related theorists shows how knowledge of theoretical perspectives can be linked to practice, while a fourth example of theory in practice shows how relatively simply adaptations or additions to service provision can make an impact on the quality of care provided.

Margaret McMillan (1860–1931)

McMillan believed that children can develop into a whole person by learning through play, and that play helps children to apply in practice what they already know and understand (Bruce and Meggitt 2002). To McMillan, relationships, feelings and ideas were as important for children as moving and learning. McMillan also believed that the play environment should be spacious and light, so that there was room to move around and play freely (Pound 2005).

The activities given to children and young people, as well as the environment they are in, need to be considered. It is well documented that children develop through play and, therefore, activities and experiences offered need to reflect this. Providing a themed imagery area allows children to act out what they know of the world around them; in a healthcare setting children may use this to help them understand and process their medical experiences. Children and young people that are in hospital should be able to use the playroom, unless they are in isolation (Chapter 8 provides an interesting case study that describes infection control issues relating to use of the playroom). In a well-planned and spacious play setting, children and young people can use the playroom in most circumstances, whether they are confined to bed, with a fractured leg in plaster, are using a wheelchair or connected to a drip stand having intravenous fluids. Careful risk assessments should make this possible, enabling the child or young person to join in with others and feel included.

Where space and the medical condition allows, toys and activities can be placed on or around the bed so that the child or young person can play. Over-the-lap trays or bedside tables can be used for painting activities, construction or board games. Electronic resources, for example, games consoles can also be used in this area.

Susan Isaacs (1885–1948)

Isaacs believed that through play children understand the world around them and that play, particularly imaginative play, can be used to help them explore their feelings. To help them develop in these areas, children should have space and freedom to move when playing.

The use of play preparation by the play specialist is a way of putting Isaac's theory into practice. Explaining to the child or young person what is going to happen, using age-appropriate language, will help them understand the procedure. They can play with a doll or soft toy, pretending to apply a bandage or use a plastic syringe and act out the procedure (Figure 5.1).

Play preparation can reduce anxiety, promote understanding and lead to discussion about what type of distraction therapy can be used during the procedure (Jun-Tai 2005). It is important that the information you give is age and stage appropriate to the child or young person. It is also important to give the child a chance to ask questions so that any misconceptions can be addressed. The information given should be factual and the amount given should be appropriate so that the child or young person is not overloaded. Being honest with the child or young person will lead to increased trust in the professional relationship, which is important if there are any future visits.

Janet Moyles

Bruce (2011) believed that children should be able to fully immerse themselves in their play. By doing this, free-flow play will take place. Bruce uses a range of characteristics to help identify play. Children should be able to choose what they

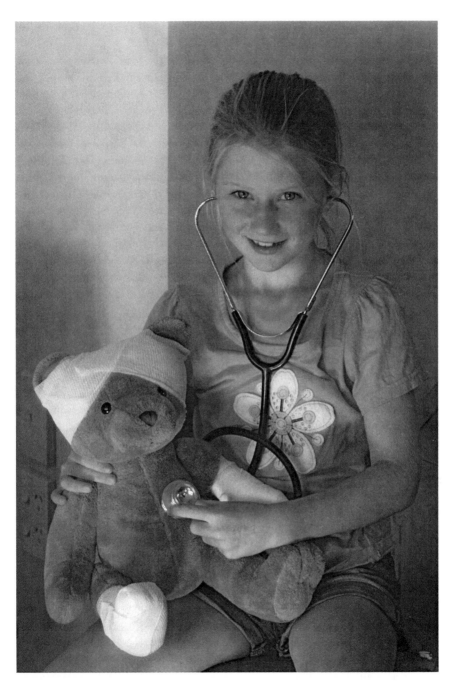

FIGURE 5.1 Preparation using real bandages and stethoscope on the child's own teddy.

play freely, use firsthand experiences and be allowed to direct their own play, making up rules and using props (Lindon 2001).

Using this information, Moyles developed the 'Play Spiral' whereby free-flow play needs to be followed by adult input which could help children to reinforce and develop their learning. Following the input of the adult, children need to be able to play freely again. An example of how you could use Moyles' play spiral is through the use of messy play, e.g. a play-dough activity. Provide play-dough, but do not put out any utensils. The child or children will explore and play with the dough. Observe how the child plays with the dough and observe interactions with other children. After a period of free-flow play, join in with the activity, but this time introduce different utensils such as a rolling pin, shape cutters and other play-dough tools. Show a child how to use the rolling pin if they are unable to do so and show them how to cut-out shapes to make 'cookies'. Introduce concepts such as size, shape and counting the cookies. Stay with the child or children for a short time, and then leave the activity for them to continue with their free-flow play. This process can be repeated when necessary, enabling a child or young person to develop skills with support from an adult.

The role of the environment

Bandura, through the concept of reciprocal determinism, described how the environment, our thinking and behaviour are constantly interchanging and the subsequent effect this has on how we feel (Pound 2005). Providing a positive environment will be beneficial for everyone. This is particularly important when operating within adult facilities.

Article 7 of the European Association for Children in Hospital (EACH) Charter states that 'children ... shall be in an environment designed, furnished, staffed and equipped to meet their needs' (EACH 2013). This is also advocated by the Department of Health (2003), who state that 'care will be provided in an appropriate location and in an environment that is safe and well suited to the age and stage of development of the child or young person'. So how can you provide an environment that is suited to the needs of children and young people?

> Having posters and glow in the dark stars in the x-ray room, colouring in pages and word searches or a small box of toys in the waiting area can help children gain a 'sense of belonging' and keep them occupied. Keeping a pot of bubbles or a flashing pen in your pocket can help to distract impatient toddlers and giving certificates after the procedure can help children leave on a positive note, which will help if future visits are needed. These resources may not be an obvious source of support for young people and it is important to remember that their needs differ (DH – Children and young people 2011). However, magazines that are appropriate for this age range may help to keep young people occupied.
>
> *(Weldon and Tonkin 2012)*

The impact of illness or health issues and the ability to play

The impact on a child or young person's ability or desire to play will vary depending on their illness or health issues. A child may have had an accident and, for example, fractured their femur and require a six-week stay in hospital, while others may need 24 hours on intravenous antibiotics for an infection. A young person may have a chronic long-term condition such as cystic fibrosis, sickle cell anaemia or cancer and may have regular visits to hospital, staying for a variable amount of time.

It is not possible to consider the impact of all the illnesses or health conditions affecting children and young people that a professional may work with, but physical, emotional and mental health factors can be evident in all of them. It is important to remember, as stated by Lindon (2002), that children who are ill still want to play and will become upset and agitated if access to play or recreational opportunities are denied.

Physical factors such as traction, restrictive splinting, plastering or drips, as well as the injury or illness itself, can make playing difficult. A child or young person may have to find alternative ways to complete tasks they can already do and thought will need to be given with regard to the positioning and type of equipment used.

Activity 5.1

Consider ways of adapting a painting activity in the following situations:

- a ten-year-old having an infusion lasting two hours;
- a six-year-old restricted to bed due to traction for a fractured femur;
- a 14-year-old who is unable to use their dominant hand.

There are many ways that barriers to play can be overcome. These will vary depending on the situation. Below are some ideas that could be used.

- Place equipment within easy reach of the child or young person. This could be on a table or bed.
- Adjust the height of the bed or table being used.
- Cover the bed, wheelchair or child or young person to prevent them getting messy.
- Use equipment with larger handles to make gripping easier.
- Use large boards or hospital tables to provide a firm surface for activities such as puzzles or drawing. Lap trays or over-the-lap tables where the height can be adjusted can be very useful.
- Use alternative equipment such as syringes when painting. The child or young person will be able to participate in the activity from further away. Paint-brushes with large or easy grip handles can also be used.

Anxiety and depression

An illness or accident may cause a child or young person to feel anxious. This can be as a result of an injury, a recent diagnosis or a long-term or terminal condition, and as a result, depression may be an issue. Anxiety and depression can affect a child or young person's interest in play. Concerns may be acted out in role-play or they may lose interest in playing altogether.

Healthcare staff should be able to help children and young people that are feeling anxious or depressed by:

- Helping children and young people to make decisions. Children and young people that are anxious or depressed may find this difficult to do. If this is the case, give children options of activities they can do, but not too many. This will enable them to make a choice without being overwhelmed with the options they are given.
- Helping children and young people make resources such as stress balls that could help them if they feel anxious.
- Enabling children and young people to 'take control' of their time and care whenever possible by letting them plan what they may want to do and when they want to do it.

Long-term conditions

A long-term condition, a long stay in hospital or recurrent visits may affect a child's social relationships with their peers, which in turn can have an effect on their ability to play. Children form friendships easily, but these may change if they cannot maintain them for a period of time. This can mean that they lose friends and therefore their playmates. Older children and young people rely heavily on the use of social media and this can bring its own difficulties (as discussed within Chapter 8). Healthcare staff can help children and young people that attend regularly by:

- encouraging children and young people to maintain communication with friends by writing letters, sending e-mails, using social media or drawing pictures;
- ensuring children and young people understand their condition or treatment process so they can explain it to friends – this may help strengthen a relationship if their friends understand what is happening;
- encouraging children and young people to attend school or complete school work so they don't fall behind.

Emergency treatment

Play can help children understand treatments and make sense of what is happening to them, prepare the child for medical procedures and offer coping strategies that make the interventions a less traumatic experience (Jun-Tai 2005). If treatment is planned, children and young people can use play to help understand and process what will take place and this can be through play preparation. For children coming into emergency departments there is no time to plan; however, play can be used before and afterwards to help them process what will or has happened. In all situations, the following suggestions may help the child or young person receiving treatment:

- Pre- and post-procedural play can be used if treatment or admission is unplanned.
- Guide children and young people to relevant literature or websites to help them and their families gain knowledge. Provide information folders and displays for children, young people and their families to look at.
- Provide equipment in the playroom, e.g. home corner that will enable children and young people to explore ideas freely.

Planned play provision

A play plan is a written record of the work carried out with an individual child or young person in a healthcare setting. It is a working document that can be added to and revised as and when needed and, importantly, it is a method of communicating with other members of the multidisciplinary team (MDT). Storing the play plan in the patient's notes allows members of the MDT to read it, providing valuable information that will help with implementing care. Play plans are an invaluable tool for measuring and recording what has happened and they can be used to help plan in the future. Play plans are written evidence for the health play specialist (HPS) and document how much work is done with individual children and young people.

Play plans show how much thought goes into providing play support to children and how much play can help facilitate recovery and promote health and emotional wellbeing. This is important as, often, the outcomes of play cannot be identified as they do not have a defined clinical outcome (Kennedy 2010).

Activity 5.2

What information needs to be recorded within a play plan?
Why is it important to include this information?

Play plans are an important and valuable way of linking theoretical perspectives and play, enabling them to be applied in practice in order to meet the holistic developmental needs of the individual children in your care. By using play plans you are taking into consideration the child's interests, likes and dislikes, age and stage of development and, importantly, their health needs.

This can be achieved by using short-term or long-term play plans. Each play plan should have a clear aim and set of objectives showing what the plan hopes to achieve for that individual, as each child or young person will have a different set of factors that need to be considered. By using play-based observations, as covered in Chapter 4, alongside information gained from the MDT, the practitioner should have a good idea of the developmental stage of the child. Cultural, emotional, ethnic, gender-based and social circumstances should be included in the planning (Gleave and Cole-Hamilton 2012). To find out the likes and dislikes of the child or young person, the practitioner can talk to them as well as involving their parents or carers in the planning. Sibling support is also important and should be included in the planning. This will help to meet the needs of the child as well as support the family.

Each hospital setting will have its own variation of play plans, and they can be tailored to suit different organizations. By capturing the information about the child, the play or activity plan not only meets the child's current needs, but can also help move them forward to facilitate progress and aid recovery.

Short-term plans can be used for children that are expected to stay in hospital or the setting for a day or so; therefore, the information included does not need to be in great detail. Long-term plans are used for those children and young people that will need re-current, longer stays. These long-term plans are useful for children and young people with conditions such as cystic fibrosis, who sometimes need lots of support to stay motivated with their treatments for a life-long condition which impacts on the family as well as the child. These plans will help to provide continuity of care as they include information from previous admissions.

It is important to allow for flexibility when planning, and plans should be adapted as needed. Plans also need to be reviewed to ensure they are working and meeting the objectives set. Play plans allow for the practitioner to reflect on what worked well or not so well. A child's mood, health problem or illness can mean that on any one day they may feel completely different from the day before and it is important to remember that what works well for one ten-year-old does not always work for another.

As a child progresses, new aims and objectives can be set. For a child receiving palliative care, sensitivity and empathy will play an important role in meeting the needs of the child or young person. Liaison with outside organizations such as respite care can be necessary and provide additional support; examples of this can be seen within Chapter 12.

Case Study 5.1

Gemma is a ten-year-old girl with cystic fibrosis. She lives with her mother and father and two older sisters. Gemma is admitted to hospital for two weeks at a time every three months and has had other regular admissions and outpatient appointments since she was diagnosed. During her admissions, she is often on her own as her parents are unable to stay on the ward, although they do visit for short periods in the day. Gemma has physiotherapy sessions three times a day, intravenous antibiotics and other potentially painful procedures.

Activity 5.3

Devise a long-term play plan for Gemma.

The HPS is in a unique position in helping to make a visit to a medical setting for a child or young person a positive experience. The HPS can look at the holistic needs of the child or young person, including their emotional needs, and use this information to plan appropriate play opportunities (Jun-Tai 2005).

The HPS is a non-threatening member of the MDT, who does not carry out any procedures or treatments on a child or young person. By gaining a child's trust and by forming professional friendships with the child or young person and their families, especially those requiring lengthy admissions or having chronic long-term conditions, the HPS can assist with many aspects of the patient's stay. The HPS can act as an advocate, speaking up for a child or young person who may be too scared, or unable, to say how they feel. The HPS can liaise between the MDT on behalf of the child or young person and their family to help achieve the best possible outcomes. The HPS role can be invaluable in offering a 'more personal' level of care and they can provide a safe, caring and nurturing environment which can make the healthcare setting a more relaxed environment for the child, young person and their family.

There are many factors that should be given thought when planning play or recreation activities for a child or young person. The patients seen in healthcare environments are from a variety of backgrounds and speak a range of languages. It is important to be respectful of the range of cultures and religions. This can be done by learning about other people's beliefs, which will help to provide equity and inclusive practice.

Children and young people, regardless of their culture, will want to play and they will find something to play with. The concept of play is consistent regardless of culture (Brown 2009). Being in hospital should therefore not be a barrier to play and recreation; play and recreation may simply need to be adapted. Children and young people requiring treatment will assume that staff understand the background they are from and their reactions (Norton and Watt 2004). Therefore, it is important to reflect the society that the child or young person lives in within the setting. Resources should reflect the ethnicity of society, not just the main ethnic groups in the local area. This will help to make the child or young person feel valued in the setting. Multicultural dolls, skin-tone paints or coloured pencils as well as dual-language books are ways in which this can be done.

Disability should not be a barrier to play (Gleave and Cole-Hamilton 2012). A child will want to play regardless of any limitations they have. A child who has multiple difficulties such as global developmental delay may enjoy playing with sensory toys or music activities and enjoy listening to stories (as described within Chapter 12). Try not to make assumptions about children who have special needs. If you are not sure about a child's condition or needs, ask someone. Talk to the child, the family or caregivers or a member of the MDT to get advice.

Activity 5.4

Consider the following questions:

If a child or young person has language difficulties, what communication methods can be used?
How could an interpreter be accessed?
What non-verbal signals could a child or young person use to try to communicate?

The importance of the multidisciplinary team

The MDT is of crucial importance in a healthcare setting. It is vital that all members work together to enable children and young people to receive the best care and treatment available. Each member has specialist knowledge, which on its own may not be enough to treat the child or young person's holistic needs.

Psycho-social meetings are held in every paediatric medical setting, usually weekly. Representatives from all parts of the MDT attend these meetings, including the health visiting team, Children's and Adolescent Mental Health Service (CAMHS), as well as safeguarding nurses, paediatric consultants, attending doctors, the nurse in charge, the ward manager or senior sister, a play specialist, school teacher, physiotherapists and any other professional who may have a concern about a particular child they want to discuss within the meeting.

Every child who has been admitted to the ward since the previous week's meeting will be discussed, and information can be shared about any social or psychological concerns. These concerns are documented by the safeguarding nurse, who will formulate a plan within the meeting and then feedback to the team in the next meeting on progress made or any other developments.

MDT meetings are essential for the sharing of information to enable the safeguarding of the children while they are within the healthcare environment and to ensure this is followed through after discharge from hospital to the community. The meetings can provide valuable information to outside agencies such as social services, schools or the child's own GP. The HPS can support the psycho-social team by attending meetings and sharing their observations from working with a child or young person.

The following information provides further insight of the importance of individual roles within an MDT, as well as how these professionals may be able to benefit from using play with children or young people.

Anaesthetists

The anaesthetic room can be a frightening experience for a child or young person. This can often be where the child or young person is most anxious and cannot have the people around them that make them feel comfortable. If the HPS accompanies the child or young person to theatre, the anaesthetist can ask them to assist with the procedures taking place. The anaesthetist can also be informed about any play preparation that has taken place and how the child has responded. This will enable them to provide a consistent approach for the patient. To make the anaesthetic room seem less frightening, mobiles or pictures can be put up for patients to look at as they are going to sleep. Operating department staff can use name badges with shapes or faces, colourful hats, bubbles and pens with lights, all of which may help the child or young person feel more relaxed.

Dieticians

Dieticians can provide advice for staff on diets for children and young people. Staff working more frequently with the child or young person may be able to provide the dietician with information about food they like or dislike. When children have a restricted diet it is important to enable them to have choices whenever possible. This could be by planning what order they want their meals in, for example a main meal at lunchtime rather than in the evening or the flavour of a drink they would like.

Healthcare staff may be able to provide reward charts, stickers or prizes for children or young people that are not complying with meal plans or are struggling to eat sufficient foods. This may motivate the child or young person to comply and to enjoy the process more. If a child with cystic fibrosis is finding it difficult to eat enough, a reward chart could be introduced. When the child complies with the eating plan they are rewarded with a sticker or stamp which they can choose. The eating plan can then be modified if necessary and after meeting the required targets, the child can be awarded a prize. It is important that the targets set are realistic and achievable or the child may become demotivated.

Doctors

The experience that doctors have of working with children can vary widely. Some will have had many years of experience and a special interest in paediatrics, while others can be new to working on a children's ward and find working with children and young people daunting. Doctors can develop their relationships with children and young people by considering their interactions with them. Kneeling down to the level of the child or young person will help the doctor seem less intimidating. Using distraction methods or asking the patient how they would like to sit or where they would like the procedure done can make the situation less stressful for all concerned. Having pens with flashing lights or asking the HPS to assist with the procedure can also help.

The HPS can offer training sessions for doctors, particularly those on rotation where this may be their first experience of working with children or young people. The training could include information on appropriate communication. For example, if a doctor tells a child they are going to take some blood, clarify how much will be taken. A pin prick may be required, but the child may imagine that a litre will be taken. The importance of child-friendly language could also be included in the training along with an awareness of the interactions with colleagues around the bed space. This is particularly important when engaging with young people who can often seem disinterested or distant when being spoken to.

The nursing team

Nurses and specialist nurses spend a lot of time with a child or young person receiving medical treatment. The majority of nurses working with children and young people will have had specialist training, but this does not necessarily mean they always find it easy or have time to play with children. Nurses can provide play equipment for the child or young person to help them stay stimulated during their stay. This could be equipment from the playroom or toys they have brought with them from home. Nurses may play games or read books with children, particularly if they are admitted for a long period of time. Nursing staff may want to use distraction equipment when changing dressings or administering drugs to help the child or young person stay calm or be more responsive.

It is important that nurses have the opportunity to contribute to play plans as they will have detailed knowledge of the child or young person. Specialist nurses can use play when working with a child or young person as a way to explore their feelings or to prepare them for a procedure or treatment that is taking place.

The HPS can assist nursing staff by helping to distract the patient during a procedure or prepare them beforehand for a procedure that is going to take place. The HPS can provide training or allow nurses to shadow them while they work with a child or young person. The HPS can leave a range of equipment for the nurses to use in the evenings, at weekends or when they are on holiday. They could also show nurses how to use the equipment or leave a list of possible activities that they could use with a child or young person.

Physiotherapists

Physiotherapy can be an important part of a child's rehabilitation and recovery. Physiotherapists can use many play techniques to encourage children or young people to participate and comply with treatment plans. It can be helpful to find out the interests of a child or young person and incorporate these into exercises they need to do, as discussed in Chapter 7. The HPS can assist physiotherapists by attending physiotherapy sessions with a child or young person, providing training or helping the child or young person do the exercises on the ward.

Radiographers

Therapeutic and diagnostic radiographers can help to make any procedures less daunting for children by considering the environment around them. They can explain to the child or young person what is going to happen during the procedure and allow them to have any support they may need, such as having parents present. However, some young people may not want their parents present, especially if the pelvic area is being X-rayed in young women of child-bearing age, when questions regarding the possibility of being pregnant need to be asked. The HPS can support a radiographer by helping to prepare a child or young person for a procedure or by attending the procedure to offer distraction while it is being carried out.

The HPS can raise awareness of their role by visiting other departments in the healthcare setting, putting up posters showing their contact details or providing training sessions. Distraction boxes can also be made by the HPS or other professionals to use with children throughout the healthcare setting.

This chapter has shown the importance of play and recreation in healthcare settings and how play can be adapted to plan for the individual needs of children and young people.

Suggested answers

Activity 5.2

These would be completed as part of the preparation:

- standard details: the child's name (be aware of confidentiality), gender, date of birth and age. If appropriate, the result of any developmental assessment undertaken;
- the date on which the play plan was devised, the diagnosis and any specific considerations that need to be taken into account;
- length of plan: short term or long term;
- aim (what you want to do) and objectives (how you are going to do it);
- proposed outcomes of the plan;
- materials and/or resources and activities to be offered.

When the play session has been completed, the following details would also be recorded:

- response to play materials or activities offered;
- interactions;
- evaluation of the play session;
- recommendations to take forward.

Activity 5.4

See Chapter 12 for an overview of how an interpreter can be used to promote play for children and young people who require assistance with accessing the language being used.

References

Brown, S. (2009) *Play: how it shapes the brain, opens the imagination, and invigorates the soul.* New York: Avery.

Bruce, T. (2011) *Learning through play: for babies, toddlers and young children*, 2nd edn, Oxon: Hodder Education.

Bruce, T. and Meggitt, C. (2002) *Child care & education*, 3rd edn, Oxon: Hodder & Stoughton.

CWDC (Children's Workforce Development Council) (2010) *The common core of skills and knowledge*, Leeds: Children's Workforce Development Council.

Department of Health (2003) *Getting the right start: National Service Framework for Children: Standard for Hospital Services.* London: Department of Health.

Department of Health – Children and Young People (2011) *You're welcome: quality criteria for young people friendly health services*, London: Department of Health.

EACH (European Association for Children in Hospital) (2013) *The 10 articles of the EACH Charter.* Online. Available: www.each-for-sick-children.org/each-charter/each-charter-and-annotations.html (accessed 13 December 2013).

Gleave, J. and Cole-Hamilton, I. (2012) *'A world without play': a literature review*, Play England.

Jun-Tai, N. (2005) *Factsheet no. 6: play in hospital.* Online. Available: www.ncb.org.uk/media/124842/no.6_play_in_hospital.pdf (accessed 13 December 2013).

Kennedy, I. (2010) *Getting it right for children and young people: overcoming cultural barriers in the NHS so as to meet their needs*, London: Department of Health.

Lindon, J. (2001) *Understanding children's play*, Cheltenham: Nelson Thornes.

Lindon, J. (2002) *Factsheet no. 3: what is play?*. Online. Available: www.ncb.org.uk/media/124824/no.3_what_is_play.pdf (accessed 13 December 2013).

NHS Employers (2010) *Appraisals and KSF made simple: a practical guide*, London: NHS Employers.

Norton, D. and Watt, S. (2004) *Transcultural health care practice with children and their families.* Online. Available: www.rcn.org.uk/development/learning/transcultural_health/transcultural/childhealth (accessed 14 December 2013).

Pound, L. (2005) *How children learn: from Montessori to Vygotsky – educational theories and approaches made easy*, Leamington Spa: Step Forward Publishing Ltd.

Unicef (2013) *Fact sheet: a summary of the rights under the Convention on the Rights of the Child.* Online. Available: www.unicef.org/crc/files/Rights_overview.pdf (accessed 13 December 2013).

Weldon, C. and Tonkin, A. (2012) How child-friendly is your department? *Synergy News*, May: 21.

6

ENHANCING RESILIENCE IN CHILDREN AND YOUNG PEOPLE

Norma Jun-Tai and Frances Barbour

This chapter will demonstrate ways in which resilience can be enhanced for children and young people. It will explore theoretical and socio-historical perspectives that have influenced and informed children's and young people's experience of being in hospital today. Attention will be given to therapeutic play interventions which promote positive emotional wellbeing for children undergoing healthcare procedures, and for their families, while recognizing that support mechanisms for practitioners are required in terms of enhancing their own resilience.

Chapter objectives

By the end of this chapter you should have an awareness of:

- the link between theory and the socio-historical perspectives that have impacted on children's and young people's experience of healthcare;
- how play can enhance resilience for children and young people;
- how consideration for the practitioner's own resilience can enhance their health and wellbeing.

THE NHS KNOWLEDGE AND SKILLS FRAMEWORK

Communication

- Shares and engages thinking with others
  - Accurate information given
  - Appropriate information given

Personal and people development

- Takes responsibility for meeting own development needs
  - People feel they have the knowledge and skills to do their jobs
  - People feel responsible for developing their own expertise

(NHS Employers 2010)

THE COMMON CORE OF SKILLS AND KNOWLEDGE

Effective communication and engagement with children, young people and families

- Summarise situations in the appropriate way for the individual (taking into account factors such as background, age and personality)
- Present genuine choices to children and young people, explaining what has happened or will happen next and what they are consenting to
- Recognise that different people have different interests in a situation and be able to work with them to reach the best and most fair conclusion for the child or young person
- Know when and how to refer to sources of information, advice or support from different agencies or professionals in children's or adult services

Child and young person development

- Encourage children or young people to value their personal experiences and knowledge
- Know how to interact with children and young people in ways that support the development of their ability to think, learn, and become independent

Multi-agency and integrated working

- Understand that others may not have the same understanding of profes-sional terms and may interpret abbreviations and acronyms differently

(CWDC 2010)

Introduction

Healthcare practitioners must be mindful that children and young people who experience healthcare interventions already exist within the context of a family and community which have, thus far, informed their education, personality and char-acteristics. In other words, they are individuals first and patients second. As dis-cussed in Chapter 3, the psychologist Uri Bronfenbrenner developed an Ecological Systems Theory (Pound 2009), which shows the child in a social context at the centre of human ecology. Bronfenbrenner argued that all systems interface and can help identify what a child needs in order to develop into a successful adult, whether it is the child's immediate family, culture, school/health needs or socio–economic conditions. Disruption to these familiar, interwoven systems can present a challenge to the way in which the child or young person successfully transitions to a new situation. Therefore, this chapter demonstrates that an understanding of how this socio–cultural perspective informs healthcare practice enables practitioners to help children and young people make sense of new and ongoing healthcare events.

The link between theory and the socio-historical perspectives

Palaiologou (2013) suggests that children learn to negotiate, problem–solve and make meaning out of their experiences through the facilitation of knowledgeable others. This process can be seen through the work of the health play specialists (HPS) who use therapeutic play techniques to scaffold the child's learning and understanding of a situation (Bruner 2006) through guided participation (Rogoff *et al.* 1993).

Activity 6.1

Review the Ecological Systems Theory proposed by Bronfenbrenner in 1979. Consider where and how your role fits in with the needs of the child and family.

- The microsystem holds the child at the centre and contains immediate caregivers.
- The mesosystem applies to the link between immediate settings and institutions, such as nursery, school, family, health services, community, place of worship.
- The exosystem relates to people or places the child does not have direct contact with, but they do have a bearing on the child's wellbeing, e.g. social/welfare services, neighbours, parents' places of work.
- The macrosystem involves the attitudes and ideologies of the culture in which the child exists, e.g. the impact of government policy, service planning and delivery.

Childhood experiences may impact on and subsequently influence our ability to cope with and overcome adversity, resulting in greater or lesser resilience to future events. Over 50 years ago, the pioneering work of Save the Children Fund and Action for Sick Children demonstrated that, in order to address a child's psychological needs in hospital, access to play and recreation and access to a familiar caregiver (Robertson 1970) are central to emotional wellbeing in this unfamiliar environment.

In 1963, Save the Children Fund employed a hospital play worker in England and, in doing so, demonstrated that play in hospital could achieve more than the relief of boredom. This model grew rapidly as doctors and nurses reported that children appeared to get better faster (OMEP 1966; Department of Health 2003). These early hospital play schemes delivered by a trained practitioner were pioneering in giving the child a voice, using therapeutic play techniques to listen to and respond to children's and young people's narratives. Today, children and young people are enabled in making sense of a potentially frightening environment through the facilitation of activities that address the 'how, why and what next' of their situation. The skilled use of coping strategies before and during painful/invasive procedures can empower children to become active rather than passive participants in terms of their own healthcare. Clark and Moss (2001) describe the 'mosaic approach' in capturing the views of children. Here, drawings, direct views, observations and responses to the environment offer important signals to the adult on how to interpret the messages the child is giving us. Appropriate action from the HPS can determine how best to respond to, and subsequently strengthen, the resilience of the children they work with. In turn, this knowledge can be synthesized to give the multidisciplinary team (MDT) a greater insight into the feelings and wishes of their patients.

Action for Sick Children drew on the significant observational work of James Robertson, Joyce Robertson, Donald Winnicott, Mary Ainsworth and John Bowlby to campaign for unrestricted access by parents to their hospitalized child, in order to uphold the need for secure attachment in early childhood. By highlighting the long-term damage that results if these attachments are broken through separation, the charity paved the way for parents to have 24-hour access to their child. Other pioneering child-centred practices were initiated, which helped children and families assimilate then accommodate new experiences, including regular visits from siblings, parents being allowed to stay overnight and parents being present during anaesthetic induction and other invasive procedures.

Garhart Mooney (2013) describes Erikson's theory of psycho-social development, entitled The Eight Ages of Man, which covers the life span of a human being. Erikson believed that, in the child's earliest years, patterns develop that regulate and influence a person's actions and interactions for the rest of their life, and depending on how we resolve issues in each stage of development, we form personality strengths and weaknesses. Although Erikson believed the early childhood years were critical in children's development of trust, autonomy and initiative, he did not believe that all was lost if children experienced difficulties early on.

As adults we understand that we are likely to experience some challenges in our lives and it is likely that early loving attachments to another person have given us the capacity to form future relationships and develop empathy and supportive networks which equip us when such situations arise. Young children have not yet made that connection and Garhart Mooney (2013: 55, 60) considers the role of adult engagement and response to a child's needs by making the link between Erikson's theory and brain development in the first 12 months of life:

> Experiences that occur within these twelve months help to determine whether a baby will wire for trust or mistrust. If a baby's needs are regularly met the baby will wire for trust. However, if a baby's needs are not regularly met it is likely to wire for mistrust but repair is still possible with the right interactions and environment ... providing meaningful, positive experiences actually alters the formation of their brains.

Goleman (2007: 185) suggests that mastery which is achieved in childhood as a result of successfully learning to cope with stresses becomes 'imprinted in their neural circuitry, leaving them more resilient when facing stress as adults'.

How play can enhance resilience for children and young people

When considering how best to help children and young people to cope in a health-care setting, an understanding of resilience and what it means for individual children will help healthcare practitioners identify and respond to the needs of the child. The term 'resilience' is defined in the Oxford Dictionaries (2013) as the capacity to recover quickly from difficulties. Hands on Scotland (2008) discusses resilience in terms of bouncing back from what life throws at us and being able to adapt well to changes and difficulties. It states that the more resilient children are, the better they cope with problems, and the better health they have.

Rutter (1981) talks of children's resilience in the face of adversity and the importance of acknowledging their perceptions of fear and personal adequacy. If the child is expected to be able to deal more effectively with fear and adequacy in later life, then healthcare practitioners have a responsibility to address their concerns at the time of treatment. The aim of the National Association of Health Play Specialists (NAHPS 2013) is to promote the physical and mental wellbeing of children and young people in hospital and community settings. Play is accepted as vital to the healthy growth and development of children. For children and young people who are undergoing a medical or surgical experience it carries greater significance. For this reason play should be a part of all children's care plans in a healthcare setting.

Case Study 6.1

A five-year-old child had been wearing spectacles for six months. She had coped well with the situation. On a visit to an eye clinic, her mother was told that her daughter would need to wear an eye patch. The healthcare professional spoke to the mother and then placed the eye patch on the child. The child left the clinic wearing the patch. She passed a mirror in the corridor and jumped when she saw her reflection. 'How will my friends know who I am Mummy?' she asked. The little girl went outside and nearly walked into a concrete pillar. At this point, the normally happy, sociable little girl pulled off her eye patch and cried inconsolably. She stated that she would never wear it again. Her mother instinctively knew that play could help her child understand better, and come through a situation which they were both finding stressful and unfamiliar. After weeks of playing together with dolls wearing eye patches, drawing and talking about eye patches, reading stories about eye patches, and family members wearing eye patches, the little girl recently went to school for the first time wearing her patch.

This child was not playing to pass time and, although she enjoyed the play very much, she was primarily using it to help her assimilate ideas, ask questions and to sort out in her own mind the reason for having to undergo this type of treatment. Unlike adults, who can rationalize and often readily understand the concept of new ideas, a young child does not have that level of developmental ability and, therefore, uses play as a way of understanding and communicating.

Barbour (2011) considers the multi-faceted nature of children's play which allows them to develop cognitively, physically and socially, and to be able to use language. As a communication tool, play affords the opportunity for young children to express themselves in a way that is often easily recognized by their peers, but is not always fully understood by adult observers. It is this lack of understanding which often leads to children's play being undervalued – regarded as something which children 'do' to pass time, or, at best, derive some pleasure from. As adults we need to continually challenge ourselves to find out what children are really saying to us, and this is particularly pertinent in healthcare settings.

According to Casey (2010), play brings many benefits in all areas of a child's being, wellbeing and development. Time spent at play is not only important for a child's social experiences, but it is also significant to the way children view the settings they spend time in, and for children with disabilities to their whole experience of inclusion.

Moyles (1989) states that 'Play is undoubtedly a means by which humans and animals explore a variety of experiences in different situations for diverse purposes' and refers to the work of Holt (1972), who suggests that children and adults all wear different 'hats' in different situations. By doing so, each grows to an understanding of the real 'self' and 'self-worth'. House (2011) draws on the work of Howard (2010), who states that children's emotional development, resilience and self-esteem are promoted by play, as it contributes to their holistic development. There is evidence of this when Milsom (1980) discusses a very ill and frightened little boy who, however unwell he became, had a daily ritual of playing tea parties with orange juice and biscuits, after which he would involve himself in a variety of different activities. Through play he was able to reassure himself that he could still do things. Even when his condition deteriorated, play was central to his needs and he continued to play tea parties, sing songs and play games.

Activity 6.2

Read the following quote:

> Psychologically play helps children cope with an uncomfortable world. If they experience something nasty they can play through the event until they feel they have mastery over it.
>
> *(Lansdown 1980: 56)*

Consider an area of your professional practice where you have observed a child playing.

- Write a brief reflective account of what you observed.
- Does access to play make a child more resilient?
- What other factors do you think can contribute to a child's resilience?

Kuttner (2010) discusses pain in children's lives, explaining that some children who report pain still wish to play, either by themselves or with others. She goes on to say that, despite the pain they are experiencing, children often want to be involved in normal daily activities by doing things that give them meaning and pleasure. It is a sign of their psychological resilience.

Recognizing the importance of resilience in healthcare settings

Young Minds (2013) suggests that, for some time, psychologists have observed that some children develop well regardless of whether they grow up in high-risk environments or not. This capacity to cope with adversity and, in some instances, be strengthened by it is at the heart of resilience. It could be argued that resilience is not something people have, but rather something they learn and, as we learn, we increase the range of strategies available to us when things become difficult.

When children, young people and their families experience trauma during medical interventions which result in symptoms of stress they may, with support, appear resilient and are, therefore, able to cope well with the situation. This group might be considered to be resilient families. Other children and families experience significant distress as a result of medically related events and situations. Their reactions can be disruptive to the way the child and family normally function and to the child or young person's medical treatment. This group might be considered to be families who struggle.

When children themselves are asked what helped them 'succeed against the odds', the most frequently mentioned facts are: help from the extended family, help from neighbours or informal mentors and positive peer relationships. No mention was made of the activities of the paid professional. Health professionals should consider this when working with children and find ways, where possible, to support and nurture relationships within the family and the wider community. Foley et al. (2001) discusses material wellbeing in terms of health, welfare and education. It is suggested that a child's own self-esteem and respect, along with the child's family and community, help promote quality of life for all children and that child care workers need to acknowledge this psycho-social agenda. If we consider that a child's wellbeing can be adversely affected in situations which are intended to promote their best interests, such as hospitalization, then a holistic approach to understanding the child's wellbeing in terms of their rights and their physical and emotional needs is required. Unicef (2013) provide information about the United Nations Convention on the Rights of the Child (UNCRC), which states that children have the same fundamental freedoms and inherent rights as all human beings, but have specific additional needs, because of their vulnerability. The concepts of vulnerability and resilience go hand in hand with two other concepts – risk factors and protective factors. Understanding risk and protective factors helps us to consider how some children cope better than others in difficult situations.

Boyden and Mann (2000), cited by Montgomery *et al.* (2003), explain that:

> Risk refers to variables that increase an individual's likelihood of psycho-pathology or their susceptibility to negative developmental outcomes. Some risks are found internally; they result from the unique combination of characteristics that make up the individual, such as temperament or neurological structure. Other risks are external; that is they result from environmental factors, such as poverty or war, which inhibits an individual's health development.

Montgomery *et al.* (2003) suggest that when children face substantial risk it is generally considered to have an impact on their health, emotions and development. Resilience can be increased through the presence of protective factors. Like risks, these protective factors can be internal or external. Internal qualities might include good health, emotional stability and adaptability, while external qualities might include adequate nutrition, environmental factors and emotionally supportive relationships.

Activity 6.3

Consider the following (fictitious) example involving two seven-year-old children, Lucy and Rachel.

Lucy is a calm child and is always willing to please. Rachel has more challenging behaviour and can be argumentative at times. Lucy's parents find their daughter a pleasure to be with and very easy-going. Rachel's parents find her difficult on occasions, and very hard to manage. Both girls are due to go into hospital for a tonsillectomy. Just before they are due to be admitted for surgery, both girls experience the death of their grandfathers. How do you think each girl might respond? How well do you think they will adjust to their hospital admission?

Now consider the following. Both girls are very fond of their grandmothers, who live in a nearby town. They have been used to visiting their grandparents once or twice a week. After the death of her husband, Lucy's grandmother decides to move to a new home about 100 miles away. At the same time, Rachel's grandmother decides to live even nearer to her granddaughter, so that she can offer extra help to the family. How do you think each child might be affected by this change in her life?

Having considered the above, and noting that the age and developmental stage of the girls, as well as their gender, will also impact on the outcome of the experiences, consider the following:

Activity 6.4

A 14-year-old male who has cystic fibrosis is admitted to the ward where you work. The young person and his family are well known to all the ward staff. The young person refuses his medication.

- Give examples of how you, as a healthcare practitioner, could work in partnership with this young person.
- Consider the wider implications of his illness on his mental wellbeing.

Applied knowledge in practice

The Department of Health (2010: 13) states that:

> We want the principles of shared decision making to become the norm: no decision about me without me. International evidence shows that involving patients in their care and treatment improves their health outcomes.

The Early Years Foundation Stage (EYFS) is the statutory framework for children from birth to five in England, which sets the standards that all early years providers must meet to ensure that children learn and develop well and are kept healthy and safe (Department for Education 2012). Within its Welfare Requirements it states that 'Children learn best when they are healthy, safe and secure, when their individual needs are met, and when they have positive relationships with the adults caring for them' (Department for Education 2012: 10). This framework is set within the context of the child's familiar routines and environment; however, as discussed, changes to this can affect a child's positive disposition to learn and develop. Health practitioners, such as play specialists, are trained to work with children in and beyond the Foundation Stage; however, the principles of providing an emotionally safe and secure environment apply across age spans. This can be seen in the National Service Framework (NSF) for Children, Young People and Maternity Services (Department of Health 2004), where therapeutic play interventions relate to most Standards, as information is presented in a culturally and age-appropriate manner supporting the process of informed consent and decision-making for children, young people and their families. When fears, anxieties and general concerns are revealed through play, timely responses can then be made by the MDT.

The following case study provides an example of how extreme fear or anxiety can be addressed. Needle phobia is often described as an intense and irrational fear produced by a specific situation, and while play specialists receive many referrals of children who have a fear of needles based on a previous negative experience, these are not always cases of phobia. However, Joe's extreme reaction to the hospital environment, which included shaking, vomiting and fainting, may have become a phobia. Being afraid of needles can cause problems for anyone, at any age. Children may not understand the medical relationship between illness and investigations, especially when they do not see themselves as sick. They, therefore, understandably question why they need to have injections or blood tests. The way the fear is handled can make a difference in building trusting relationships with medical personnel and future compliance. Adolescents who hold intense fear or phobias around needle interventions often suffer additional conflicts of emotion through the embarrassment of going for a test that has to be abandoned because the fear is just too much to cope with.

Case Study 6.2

Read the case study and consider how the HPS supported the young person in his ability to regain control over a stressful period in his life, and offer strategies for future healthcare procedures.

Joe is 14 years old and has had some negative experiences in the past surrounding blood tests and hospitals in general. He is being treated for a condition which requires a blood test every three weeks, in order to assess the level of medication required. Joe was referred by a consultant paediatrician to the play specialist following his first blood test appointment, which left him shaking, upset and embarrassed on the floor of the paediatric phlebotomist's room.

Objective

To offer coping strategies that will enable him to cooperate with the procedure of venepuncture and to use the chosen method as a resource for future invasive procedures, in order to minimize the intense fear and anxiety he experienced.

Method

Joe's first session began with some general discussion to help put him at ease and to provide the HPS with some background information, including his likes and dislikes and any hobbies/interests he may have. During this session the HPS introduced the idea of using guided imagery as a possible technique in addressing his fear of needles, and he was keen to explore this option. Guided imagery involves the patient constructing an image in their mind and then entering that scene before the procedure commences. Joe decided that his subject would be his favourite football team, as he occasionally goes to matches. The HPS would begin the session with some general relaxation exercises, then guide him through a match day from going on the train, into the stadium, watching the game and going home again. The guided imagery included thinking about sounds, smells and feelings that would be associated with the football match.

Overview of the sessions

After the initial practice of guided imagery, Joe said he felt confident that it went well and he left feeling happy and positive. A further appointment was arranged, but this time it was explained that another HPS would be present and the process of graduated exposure would begin, which involved placing the tourniquet around his arm for a few seconds and holding it as though he was having the blood test while participating in guided imagery. It was important for Joe to have complete trust in the HPS and be reassured that this would be a practice session and no procedure involving needles would take place.

At his session Joe confidently informed the HPS that he had practised his breathing/relaxation exercises and was still happy to have the tourniquet put on during the guided imagery: his football team would continue to be the focus of the imagery. When the practice session was over, Joe opened his eyes and commented that the tourniquet had not felt as tight as it had previously, because he felt so relaxed. The HPS asked if he would feel confident in having a blood test now, using the guided imagery technique, and he replied that he would like one more practice just to be sure.

Outcome

The following week, Joe had Ametop cream applied at home by his mother, to minimize the waiting time in the hospital, as he felt this added to his anxiety; in response to this, when Joe arrived those involved in the procedure were ready to do the test. The HPS began the relaxation process and then guided Joe into the football match. Once he was totally relaxed and engaged, the phlebotomist proceeded with the blood test. The test was carried out successfully and Joe was extremely pleased with the outcome. Since then he has had two more blood tests and has coped well with each one. During the last blood test, Joe felt confident enough to decline the offer of Ametop and relied solely on Ethyl Chloride spray and guided imagery. This technique is now in place for all his blood tests.

How consideration for the practitioner's own resilience can enhance their health and wellbeing

'The general public expects to be cared for by staff with the right skills and qualifications to do their jobs properly' (NAHPS 2013), but what about those doing the caring?

Healthcare practitioners, such as play specialists, use non–directive play approaches to tune in to patients. This means allowing the child to lead the play while drawing on adult-initiated skills to really help the child or young person make sense of new situations. This requires competent use of questioning and observation techniques, along with intuitive responses, in order to be effective in giving the child a voice with which to express his/her anxieties or understanding of events. This is essential front line work but, compared to other health professionals, play staff may not always receive validation of their role (Kennedy 2010) due to the number employed across NHS Trusts. Whatever our professional role, we all need affirmation from those we work alongside in order to remain positive and feel valued. Maslow's hierarchy of needs is a reminder that when lower-order needs, such as physical, physiological, safety and psychological factors have been successfully met, humans can be fulfilled through esteem needs, i.e. feeling achievement, responsibility, reputation, through to self-actualizing needs – becoming all that one is capable of becoming (Johnson 2010).

Daniel Goleman recognized that emotional intelligence is relevant to organizational development and in developing people. It provides ways to understand and assess people's behaviours, management styles, attitudes, interpersonal skills and potential (Chapman 2000). Goleman identified the five 'domains' of emotional intelligence as:

1 knowing your emotions
2 managing your own emotions
3 motivating yourself
4 recognizing and understanding other people's emotions
5 managing relationships, i.e. managing the emotions of others

(Chapman 2012)

Therefore, a greater awareness and application of these domains in yourself may equip you with the professionalism required for the challenges of daily practice.

Healthcare practitioners can experience a range of emotions in one day. The natural effervescence shared by staff, children and young people in a paediatric setting can be overshadowed by parental anxiety or the inevitable sadness when a child dies or is admitted with life-threatening/complex needs. Working as part of an MDT should provide practitioners with a joint sense of community; however, this is not always a shared perception. Miller and Cable (2010) consider Wenger's (1998) views on the way professionals from different training routes and practices construct their identities when working together, which may be based on their own professional language and perspective. By engaging in opportunities to utilize different skill sets in order to achieve a common goal, we are in a stronger position to not only offer holistic care to our patients, but also to counter stress by experiencing higher levels of satisfaction in our working life.

Additional stress factors exist for lone practitioners, such as play specialists who may be based in busy environments and experience workload dilemmas – for example, knowing that they won't be able to work with the children in isolation cubicles because the preparation and distraction of anxious or uncooperative children during invasive procedures have become a priority. Burnard (1991: 6) uses an interesting metaphor to capture a situation in which work pressures and limited time 'relates to a person rescuing people from a raging river but being unable to stop and go further up the river to see what is causing the people to fall in'.

Bailey and Clarke (1989) discuss the Transactional Model of Stress as one model which acknowledges that an individual's perception of a situation plays a large part in determining whether or not the situation is stressful. This model suggests that stress is psychological rather than physiological, as individual responses will vary according to their history, expectations and previous experience.

Perhaps a key message in responding to stress is to know your options. Bond and Holland (1998: 17) cite Proctor (1986) in the context of clinical supervision. Supervision is defined as 'a way of supporting workers who are affected by the distress, pain and fragmentation of the client and how they need time to become aware of how this has affected them and how to deal with reactions'.

Activity 6.5

Look again at Goleman's five domains.

- Use each heading to make a list of the resources you can draw on to strengthen your own sense of resilience.

Suggested answers to activities

Activity 6.1

Q. Consider where and how your role fits in with the needs of the child and family
A. Possible answers could include:

- being respectful of the wider socio-cultural norms in which the child exists;
- working collaboratively with the multidisciplinary and multi-agency teams;
- recognizing that play and leisure activities can reveal insightful perspectives from the child and young person, therefore responding appropriately to this information in order to support accurate care plans

Activity 6.2

Q. Does access to play help to make a child more resilient? If yes, in what way?
A. Possible answers could include:

- mastery over a situation;
- confidence building;

- making new relationships;
- opportunities for new experiences;
- building of communication skills;
- increased self-esteem and sense of worth.

Q. What other factors do you think can contribute to a child's resilience?
A. Possible answers could include:

- age and stage of development;
- gender;
- socio-economic factors;
- culture;
- personality;
- family characteristics;
- exposure to success in handling adversity;
- environment;
- good health.

Activity 6.3

This activity is designed to illustrate the way risk and protective factors are part of children's vulnerability or resilience. Admission to hospital might be considered an external risk to the wellbeing of both girls. Lucy's calm disposition might allow her to cope better than Rachel in the situation. However, the death of their grandfathers could be viewed as an internal risk for both girls. Risk cannot be viewed in isolation. It interacts with other risks and protective factors. If Lucy's grandmother moves away, this would be an additional external factor that might affect her wellbeing. Rachel's wellbeing might be increased if her grandmother moves nearer to the family home.

Activity 6.4

Q. Give examples of how you as a healthcare practitioner could work in partnership with this young person.
A. Possible answers might include:

- respecting differing views;
- building a trusting relationship;
- listening;
- creating a caring environment;
- working with others.

Q. Consider the wider implications of his illness on his mental wellbeing.
A. Possible answers might include:

- poor self-esteem;
- peer group pressure;
- poor educational attainment;
- lack of confidence and self-worth;
- difficulty in building and sustaining relationships.

Activity 6.5

Q. Daniel Goleman's five domains: use each heading to make a list of the resources you can draw on to strengthen your own sense of resilience.
A. Possible answers could include:

- managing your time;
- annual/bi-annual professional development planning meetings – PDP;
- meetings with mentors;
- regular access to CPD activities;
- clinical supervision;
- maintaining professional boundaries;
- joining your professional association;
- not being afraid to ask for help or advice from your appropriate professional lead;
- making time for positive experiences away from work;
- remaining up-to-date and competent to practice through professional registration.

Useful sources of further information

Action for Sick Children: www.actionforsickchildren.org.uk
Action for Sick Children: Scotland www.ascscotland.org.uk
Child and Adolescent Mental Health: www.camh.org.uk
Cruse Bereavement Care: www.crusebereavementcare.org.uk
Cruse Bereavement Care Scotland: www.crusescotland.org.uk
Cruse Young Person's helpline – for bereaved adolescents and persons: www.RD4U.org.uk
Mental Health Foundation: www.mentalhealth.org.uk
Mind: www.mind.org.uk
Winston's Wish – for bereaved children and families: www.winstonswish.org.uk

References

Bailey, R. and Clarke, M. (1989) *Stress and coping in nursing*, London: Chapman and Hall Ltd.
Barbour, F. (2011) Play in healthcare settings. *First Five: The Magazine of the Scottish Pre-School Association*, Summer: 12–13.
Bond, M. and Holland, S. (1998) *Skills of clinical supervision for nurses*, Buckingham: Open University Press.

Bruner, J.S. (2006) *In Search of Pedagogy Volume II: The Selected Works of Jerome Bruner, 1979–2006*, Oxon: Routledge.

Burnard, P. (1991) *Coping with stress in the health professions: a practical guide*, London: Chapman and Hall.

Casey, T. (2010) *Inclusive play: practical strategies for children from birth to eight*, 2nd edn, London: Sage Publications.

Chapman, A. (2012) *Emotional intelligence (EQ)*. Online. Available: www.businessballs.com/eq.htm (accessed 15 December 2013).

Clark, A. and Moss, P. (2001) *Listening to young children: the mosaic approach*, London: National Children's Bureau.

CWDC (Children's Workforce Development Council) (2010) *The common core of skills and knowledge*, Leeds: Children's Workforce Development Council.

Department for Education (2012) *Statutory Framework for the Early Years Foundation Stage*. Online. Available: www.education.gov.uk/publications/standard/AllPublications/Page1/DFE-00023-2012 (accessed 15 December 2013).

Department of Health (2003) *Getting the Right Start: National Service Framework for Children, Standard for Hospitals*, London: Department of Health.

Department of Health (2004) *National service framework: children, young people and maternity services*. Online. Available: www.gov.uk/government/publications/national-service-framework-children-young-people-and-maternity-services (accessed 15 December 2013).

Department of Health (2010) *Equity and excellence: liberating the NHS*, Norwich: The Stationery Office.

Foley, P., Roche, J. and Tucker, S. (eds) (2001) *Children in society: contemporary theory, policy and practice*, London: Palgrave Macmillan.

Garhart Mooney, C. (2013) *Theories of childhood: an introduction to Dewey, Montessori, Erikson, Piaget and Vygotsky*, 2nd edn, St. Paul, MN: Redleaf Press.

Goleman, D. (2007) *Social intelligence*, London: Arrow Books.

Hands on Scotland (2008) *Resilience*. Online. Available: www.handsonscotland.co.uk/flourishing_and_wellbeing_in_children_and_young_people/resilience/resilience.html (accessed 15 December 2013).

House, R. (2011) *Too much, too soon? Early learning and the erosion of childhood*, Gloucestershire: Hawthorn Press.

Johnson, J. (2010) *Positive and trusting relationships with children in early years settings*, Exeter: Learning Matters.

Kennedy, I. (2010) *Getting it right for children and young people: overcoming cultural barriers in the NHS so as to meet their needs*, London: Department of Health.

Kuttner, L. (2010) *A child in pain: what health professionals can do to help*, Carmarthen: Crown House Publishing Ltd.

Lansdown, R. (1980) *More than sympathy*, London: Tavistock Publications.

Miller, L. and Cable, C. (eds) (2010) *Professionalization, leadership and management in the early years*, London: Sage Publications.

Milsom, J. (1980) Spotlight on children, the hospital play specialist. *Nursing Times*, 6 March: 8.

Montgomery, H., Burr, R. and Woodhead, M. (eds) (2003) *Changing childhoods: local and global*, Milton Keynes: Open University Press

Moyles, J.R. (1989) *Just Playing? The Role and Status of Play in Early Childhood Education*, Milton Keynes: Open University Press.

NAHPS (National Association of Health Play Specialists) (2013) *National occupational standards*. Online. Available: www.nahps.org.uk (accessed 15 December 2013).

NHS Employers (2010) *Appraisals and KSF made simple: a practical guide*, London: NHS Employers.

OMEP (1966) *Play in hospital*, London: Housing Centre Trust.

Oxford Dictionaries (2013) *Definition of 'resilience' in English*. Online. Available: www.oxforddictionaries.com/definition/english/resilience?q=resilience (accessed 15 December 2013).

Palaiologou, L. (ed.) (2013) *The Early Years Foundation Stage theory and practice*, London: Sage Publications.

Pound, L. (2009) *How children learn 3: contemporary thinking and theorists*, London: Practical Pre-School Books.

Robertson, J. (1970) *Young children in hospital*, London: Tavistock Publications.

Rogoff, B., Mosier, C., Mistry, J. and Goncu, A. (1993) Toddlers' guided participation with their caregivers in cultural activity. In Forman, E., Minick, N. and Stone, A. (eds), *Contexts for learning: sociocultural dynamics in children's development*, New York: Oxford University Press.

Rutter, M. (1981) *Maternal deprivation reassessed*, 2nd edn, London: Penguin Books Ltd.

Unicef (2013) *Conventions on the Rights of the Child*. Online. Available: www.unicef.org/crc (accessed 15 December 2013).

Young Minds (2013) *Young minds in schools: risk and resilience*. Online. Available: www.youngminds.org.uk/training_services/young_minds_in_schools/wellbeing/risk_and_resilience (accessed 15 December 2013).

7

PROMOTING HEALTH AND WELLBEING

Alison Tonkin and Jenni Etchells

This chapter will explore the use of play and recreation in the healthcare setting for developing, maintaining and promoting the health and wellbeing of children and young people. Examples of how play and recreation contribute to health and wellbeing within healthcare delivery are embedded within the chapter content.

Chapter objectives

By the end of this chapter you should be able to:

- define the concepts of health and wellbeing in relation to children and young people;
- acknowledge the importance of play and recreation for children and young people's holistic health and wellbeing when used in healthcare practice;
- relate practical approaches to promoting health and wellbeing with children and young people according to their individual lifestyles and experiences.

THE NHS KNOWLEDGE AND SKILLS FRAMEWORK

Communication

- Uses a range of communication channels to build relationships
- Shares and engages thinking with others

Service improvement

- Enables and encourages others to suggest change, challenge tradition and share good practice with other areas of the trust

(NHS Employers 2010)

THE COMMON CORE OF SKILLS AND KNOWLEDGE

Effective communication and engagement with children, young people and families

- Be self aware. Know how to demonstrate a commitment to treating all people fairly, be respectful by actively listening and avoiding assumptions. Make sure your actions support the equality, diversity, rights and responsibilities of children, young people, their parents and carers

Child and young person development

- Encourage children or young people to value their personal experiences and knowledge
- Understand that play and recreation that is directed by babies, children and young people – rather than by adults – has a major role in helping them to understand themselves and the world. It also helps them to build confidence and realise their potential
- Understand the impact of technology on children and young people's lives

(CWDC 2010)

Introduction

Health and wellbeing are multidimensional concepts that are influenced by many factors. There are many different avenues that could have been explored within a chapter of this nature, but many have links with topics that are covered elsewhere in this book. For example, enhancing resilience which contributes to emotional wellbeing and mental health is covered within Chapter 6, while actively engaging children and young people in the design and delivery of health services, which enhances mental health and wellbeing, is covered within Chapter 10.

Gleave and Cole-Hamilton (2012: 22) suggest 'A world that understands and supports children's play is a world that is likely to be healthier, more vital, more alive and happier than a world without play.' Therefore, this chapter focuses on how the use of play and recreational activities and resources can be used to enhance the health and wellbeing of children and young people who come into contact with health-related services.

Defining health

Health is considered to be a dynamic concept that is constantly changing (Jack and Holt 2008). The universal definition from the World Health Organization (WHO) has not been amended since 1948, defining health as 'a state of complete physical,

mental and social wellbeing and not merely the absence of disease or infirmity'
(World Health Organization 2003a). However, Bruce and Meggitt (2005) suggest
that health needs to be viewed as a more holistic concept, adding emotional, spiritual and environmental health as important aspects that should also be considered.
Ewles and Simnett (2003) also promote a holistic approach but describe dimensions
as opposed to aspects and have incorporated environmental health into a societal
dimension, showing how society as opposed to the individual influences services,
facilities and attitudes that contribute to a healthy lifestyle. Table 7.1 summarizes
the holistic approach to health and some of the considerations you may like to
explore when working with children and young people accessing healthcare facilities and services.

TABLE 7.1 Holistic overview of health

Aspect	Description	Considerations
Physical	How the body functions	Effect of long-term or acute conditions on normal functioning
Social	Interacting and relating with other people ... forming and maintaining friendships and relationships	Effect of visiting restrictions or the isolating effects of illness and subsequent treatment regimes
Mental	The organization of thoughts and being able to think clearly	Closely linked to emotional and social health and the concept of wellbeing
Emotional	The expression of emotions and being able to deal with thoughts and feelings, e.g. fear, frustration, happiness	Resilience and the development of coping strategies. Being able to facilitate expression of emotions throughout the healthcare journey
Spiritual	Associated with a quest for 'inner peace' and personal principles and conduct	Influenced by nature and the natural world – can be linked to 'awe and wonder' and is very personal to the individual
Environmental	Factors linked to the environment which influence the health of individuals, e.g. pollution or social housing conditions	Often beyond the control of the individual, requiring society to act on behalf of the individual
Societal	Incorporates environmental health but also includes society's 'moulding' of health-related attitudes and behaviour, e.g. a ban on smoking in public places 'nudges' people to do things differently	Seen as a reflection of the society in which people live, e.g. intolerance or fear of children playing outside can limit opportunities for physical activity

Source: adapted from Bruce and Meggitt 2005; Ewles and Simnett 2003.

The inclusion of societal health is particularly important at a time when the government's public health agenda is placing increasing emphasis on the individual's ability to make informed choices about their health and to be able to cope with the impact of illness (GOV.UK 2013c). Although this is predominantly targeted towards adult services, there is a growing awareness of the need to actively encourage children and young people to use their experiences and expertise of health service utilization as drivers for change (Department of Health – Children and Young People 2011). As part of this process, the role of play and recreation is becoming more prominent, particularly in relation to wellbeing and mental health (Play England 2008).

Activity 7.1

Take one activity that links to promoting health, e.g. physical activity or enabling young people to use social media while staying in hospital.

- Identify how many different aspects of health can be linked to your one activity.
- How could you use this information when planning health-related activities with children and/or young people in a healthcare setting?

Physical activity has obvious benefits for health because the impact can be measured through specific links to the functioning of the body. For example, it can improve cardiovascular and bone health, is important for maintaining a healthy weight and it develops movement and coordination (GOV.UK 2013a). All children and young people should have the opportunity to take part in physical activities. Healthcare professionals have a key role in the facilitation of this for children and young people who may be restricted by physical limitations due to their condition. Children and young people with long-term conditions can face barriers when engaging in physical activities and there may be some physical activities that are inappropriate. For example, children and young people with cystic fibrosis who have an enlarged spleen or diseased liver should avoid contact or collision sports (Philpott *et al.* 2010). Careful consideration by the multidisciplinary team (MDT) and a coordinated approach should ensure that physical activity is safe and an individual's 'unique exercise tolerance and physical capacity' is accounted for (Philpott *et al.* 2010).

Similarly, children and young people with physical disabilities such as cerebral palsy have barriers to physical activity, yet the benefits of physical activities are inclusive to all children. To overcome this, the use of new technologies is enabling new forms of physical activity to be undertaken. Preliminary results from a collaborative research project undertaken by Sussex Community NHS Trust, Guy's and St Thomas' NHS Trust and academics at Goldsmiths, University of London and Oxford Brookes University have shown the benefit of using the Nintendo Wii Fit for children with motor difficulties. The positive physical outcomes also led to enhanced social and emotional outcomes for the children involved (Oxford Brookes University 2013). Practical solutions such as wheelchair adaptations ensure a child or young person is safe when participating in physical activity. This may need to be reviewed by the occupational therapist. Care plans to facilitate physical activity within a school setting may be written or reviewed alongside the child and their parents, the physiotherapist and children's community nurse and/or school nurse. Healthcare professionals may also enable access for children and young people to appropriate community-based fitness professionals. This demonstrates how a collaborative effort may be required to ensure that children and young people, regardless of their health status or disability, can still partake in physical activity, thereby increasing their sense of wellbeing.

Policy such as the Olympic and Paralympic legacy is important for providing motivation for physical activity across society. One of three main themes to have emerged following the Olympics and Paralympics is the commitment to the provision of support and opportunities to participate in sport and physical activities for all (GOV.UK 2013b). Broadcasting of Paralympic events may also give children and young people a 'can do' attitude that can motivate and inspire them to ensure their opportunities are not limited by their physical condition. Positive role modelling from athletes who have a disability could also help to encourage children and young people to overcome barriers and ensure that they are supported to develop and maintain healthy behaviours.

As shown above, engaging in physical activity has a positive influence on other aspects of health, particularly when linked to the outdoor world. Play England (2013) is a founding member of 'The wild network', which has been launched to try to 'reverse the trend of children losing touch with the natural world and playing outdoors'. Spirituality is strongly associated with the natural world (The Scout Association 2012) and the influence of nature is increasingly being factored into healthcare delivery and design. The extensive use of natural light has been highlighted as a unique feature of the new £100 million University College Hospital Macmillan Cancer Centre in a built-up area of central London, which also includes a rooftop garden that is available for everyone to enjoy (University College London Hospitals 2013). Play Wales (2012) advocate that 'planning and development of hospitals grounds, wards, staff childcare settings, clinics and surgeries should include comprehensive access to indoor and outdoor play provision'. Leicester Royal Infirmary has a play roof that can be accessed in all weather, enabling children who are constantly indoors on the ward access to fresh air and a change of scenery (BBC News 2008).

The influence of nature can also be reflected positively within the clinical environment. Acknowledging Bandura's theory of reciprocal determinism, the way we feel is constantly changing as a result of interactions between the environment, our thinking and behaviour (Allen and Gordon 2011). This clearly suggests that the environment plays a significant role in how children and young people feel when coming into healthcare settings. For the new Children's Unit at Salisbury District

Hospital, 'themes based on the natural environment were chosen to help reduce the usual clinical atmosphere of the hospital building' (Bayliss Robbins 2012). This unit was designed with children and young people, reflecting their needs and identities, both of which contribute to the holistic promotion of health.

Over the past decade mental health has become an increasing priority for the government, with figures now showing that 10 per cent of children aged 5 to 16 years have a diagnosable mental health problem (NHS Confederation 2012). Not only is mental health associated with poor physical health (Department of Health 2013), but many people with a long-term condition are also reported to have a mental health problem (Naylor *et al.* 2012). Mental health affects all features of a child's development, impacting directly upon a child or young person's quality of life. Early identification and intervention is vital as childhood experiences lay down developmental patterns for future mental health (Young Minds 2013b). Some practical tasks that every healthcare professional can promote on a daily basis to enhance mental health capacity are encouragement to eat well, facilitating exercise and taking time out to talk to friends and family about stressful situations (Young Minds 2013a). This may have no bearing on the known environmental or societal influences that have been shown to have negative effects on children and young people's mental health. However, any activity that benefits a child or young person's wellbeing should never be undermined, however simple it may appear. The Mental Health Implementation Framework (Department of Health 2013) has highlighted the importance of a multi-agency commitment to ensuring that mental health is improved, following on from the cross-government outcomes strategy 'No health without mental health' (Her Majesty's Government and Department of Health 2011). Early intervention and integrated support are outlined as key strategies, while mental health service improvement has been identified as an early priority for Clinical Commissioning Groups (CCG). An awareness of the professional roles and services available to support mental health should be acknowledged and professionals should always refer children and young people onto specialist services such as Child and Adolescent Mental Health Services (CAMHS) where indicated.

Defining wellbeing

Many of the domains associated with wellbeing are mirrored in the aspects and dimensions of health discussed above. However, wellbeing changes throughout the life course and is strongly associated with a person's quality of life (Fauth 2008). Wellbeing can therefore be seen as dynamic and multifactorial, encompassing both objective and subjective measurements (Carter 2012). Objective measurements have traditionally been used to 'quantify' wellbeing but these tended to rely on adult perceptions of what constitutes wellbeing for children and young people (The Children's Society 2012). Objective aspects focus on things that affect children's feelings and these are often things that may not be controlled by the child or young person themselves, e.g. poverty, housing, education and health (Carter 2012). Although adult assumptions may accurately identify the key features that influence children's wellbeing, they do not necessarily reflect the significance attached to these features and, as a result, their importance may be overlooked (The Children's Society n.d.). Indeed, one of the key recommendations for the government from Unicef following the comparative review of wellbeing in rich countries was that they should 'ask children how they feel about their lives' (Unicef United Kingdom 2013).

The Children's Society, in collaboration with the University of York, has collated substantial data since 2005 about wellbeing directly from the voices of children and young people in the United Kingdom. Their ongoing research provides a collection of qualitative accounts, with most recent research giving a voice to younger children and their unique perception of wellbeing.

Activity 7.2

According to the Good Childhood Index published in 2010 by The Children's Society (2012), the following ten areas were explored with children and young people in relation to their overall wellbeing. They are in no particular order.

1 family
2 home
3 money and possessions
4 friendships
5 school
6 health
7 appearance
8 time use
9 choice and autonomy
10 the future

- How do you think priorities may differ according to the child's or young person's age?
- How do you think priorities may differ according to a child's or young person's health status?

According to Public Health England (2013), children and young people can make the link between wellbeing and health-related behaviour and 84 per cent of children rated their health as being 'good' or 'very good'. La Valle and Payne (2012) state that children and young people readily acknowledge the importance of being healthy. However, they also suggest that for children who view their health as being 'very bad', they are more likely to be unhappy with their lives as a whole. This poses a challenge to those in the healthcare sector because coordination of care to effectively manage the holistic aspects of health also needs to address wellbeing as a whole.

Why is promoting the role of play and recreation important for health and wellbeing?

According to the *Charter for Children's Play* (Play England 2009), children who experience discomfort, anxiety or fear as a result of visiting unfamiliar or controlled environments such as hospitals may need additional support if they are to exercise their right to play. Play is an innate activity which arises out of evolutionary traits that contribute to healthy development and wellbeing (Gleave and Cole-Hamilton 2012). As such, it is recognized that all children and young people need to play, although enabling play to occur sometimes needs facilitation and support (Skills Active 2013c).

In 2008 Play England published a policy briefing entitled 'Play and health: making the link', outlining why play is 'crucial to children's healthy development and happiness' (Play England 2008). This explicitly makes a connection between play and children's health and wellbeing, particularly in relation to emotional strength and mental health, both of which require additional support when children and young people have a long-term illness or are acutely unwell. When considering health and wellbeing holistically, Play Wales (2012) suggest 'facilitating opportunities for play in hospitals:

- create an environment where stress and anxiety are reduced
- helps the child regain confidence and self esteem
- provides an outlet for feelings of anger and frustration
- helps the child understand treatment and illness.'

The Royal College of Nursing (2011) advocate that all children visiting or staying in hospital have a basic need for play and recreation that should be used as a child-centred communication tool. This should be encouraged throughout the MDT and is a powerful way of accessing children's and young people's feelings and understanding about what is happening in a secure and non-threatening manner. The International Network of Health Promoting Hospitals and Health Services (2012) have provided an assessment tool for health professionals that enable the evaluation of play and learning within hospitals and health settings. The emphasis is predominantly on play as a structured activity with a purpose, often relating to a clinical outcome. Cole-Hamilton identifies the dangers of losing sight of play as an intrinsically motivated behaviour, which is undertaken by children and young people themselves, for themselves, following their own ideas and in their own time (Gleave and Cole-Hamilton 2012). Play England (2008) emphasizes the need for health professionals to understand and recognize the role of play provision, particularly free-flow play that is child centred and child initiated. Access to unstructured, child-initiated play is increasingly being seen as fundamental to children's physical, emotional and psychological wellbeing (Cole-Hamilton and Gleave, 2011).

Free-flow play within the early years was framed as a concept by Tina Bruce, who noted that 'children's play is at its richest when they are able to "wallow" in it' (Pound 2009). Bruce (2011) identified 12 features of free-flow play and although these are generally linked to various aspects of children's development, particularly how children learn, they can be useful for guiding adults in play facilitation.

Activity 7.3

The Royal National Institute for the Blind (2011) have adapted the '12 features of play' to produce an Effective Practice Guide that can be accessed via www.rnib.org.uk/professionals/Documents/plannedplay.doc

- Review the 12 features of play and reflect on *how* each feature has been adapted to facilitate free play for a child who is visually impaired.
- Identify one aspect of provision that you offer linked to health and explore ways in which you could facilitate a less structured approach to play provision.

The importance of providing free-flow play opportunities for young children is well documented and is embedded within the Early Years Foundation Stage (Early Education 2012). The adaptation of play opportunities, as explored within Activity 7.3, demonstrates how facilitation of play 'alongside play that is designed to improve children's understanding of their condition and medical procedures can enhance their overall health and wellbeing' (Play Wales 2012). However, this is equally important for older children and young people, although the adaptations and needs of young people may not be the same (Skills Active 2013a).

Although playwork is seen as a distinct area of practice, the key principles underpinning practice (Playwork Principles Scrutiny Group Cardiff 2005) can be utilized within healthcare settings. Recognizing that health workers will use play for different purposes, the playwork sector is keen to engage with other professionals in order to share their professional knowledge (Skills Active 2013b). While acknowledging the need for healthcare professionals to undertake investigations, develop interventions and promote compliance with treatment regimes is their primary focus, it is important to remember that other aspects of children's and young people's care also need to be considered:

> For playworkers, the play process takes precedence and playworkers act as advocates for play when engaging with adult agendas.
>
> *(Skills Active 2013a)*

This has been reflected through the adoption of the Nintendo Wii as a therapeutic aid in physiotherapy programmes, which was first reported in 2009 as part of a rehabilitation programme for amputees. Used as part of the physiotherapy routine 'after their normal exercises they hop onto the Wii so that they can have some fun, but also work on their muscles and improve their balance' (CBBC Newsround 2009).

HPSs are uniquely positioned within the healthcare sector to lead 'playful activities' as well as using play as a therapeutic tool (NHS Careers 2013). Although the role of the HPS is often associated with therapeutic interventions such as preparation, distraction and post-procedural play, the ethos that underpins practice is 'the provision of recreational outlets and fun activities in the clinical environment' (Hospital Play Staff Education Trust 2013). In order to do this, the HPS has to have a sound knowledge and understanding of the role of play, particularly in relation to sick children, young people and their families (Hubbuck 2009). The HPS knows the value of play and how this can link to promoting the holistic health and wellbeing of the child or young person. For example, children's subjective views of happiness are associated with 'being able to do what they want, when they want to do it' (Cole-Hamilton and Gleave 2011) and this is particularly important as children get older, when choice and autonomy are crucial for mental health and overall wellbeing (The Children's Society 2012).

Promoting health and wellbeing with children and young people as service users

Bruce (2011: 84) states that 'Play opens up new possibilities in thinking and develops the emotional intelligence to make feelings manageable.'

Research conducted by Aldiss *et al.* (2009) explored young children's experiences of cancer care services and found that a crucial part of the hospital experience was play. Young children can be helped to understand what is happening when they use health-related services, although the NHS Confederation (2012) state that this is 'seldom mentioned by health professionals and others'.

Understanding the needs and requirements of young people accessing and engaging with health services is imperative to enable them to become lifelong health service users (Department of Health – Children and Young People 2011). The WHO regard adolescent health as a global public health issue, stating that barriers must be overcome to ensure that young people obtain the health services they require, in a way that is responsive to their individual needs (World Health Organization 2013). Although neither play nor recreation are specifically mentioned, the WHO state that services need to be appropriate and acceptable. Care must be taken to do this in conjunction with the young person as there is evidence to suggest that although healthcare services tick the boxes for being accessible and available, this does not necessarily mean that they are accepted (Tylee *et al.* 2007).

Listening and responding to children and young people's views is frequently acknowledged as best practice and this is covered in detail in Chapter 10. A joint report by the Royal College of Paediatric and Child Health and the NHS Confederation (2011) highlights the importance of health services empowering children and young people to feel valued, which subsequently enhances their wellbeing. After years of campaigning by young people and health practitioners alike, young people are now being given personal space that is tailored to their individual needs and preferences (Hutton 2010). Ideally, routines that reflect the differing nature of sleep and eating patterns should also be considered when considering health holisti-cally. The provision of 'cook to order' food on paediatric oncology wards has been shown to enable children and young people to eat when they want as opposed to the need to comply with standard meal rounds, resulting in less waste and improved nutritional support (Houlston *et al.* 2009). This highlights the importance of young people being able to demonstrate to the healthcare team what is important to them (Hutton 2010), thereby enabling young people to be cared for as a distinct group in a manner that reflects their needs and priorities. As a result, young people who feel valued and have a trusting relationship with healthcare staff will feel supported, which enhances their emotional health and wellbeing.

Globally, it is agreed that children and young people with long-term conditions often have poor compliance with treatment regimes (Dawood *et al.* 2010). There is a growing emphasis on the concept of self-care within the adult health policy agenda, but recommendations have also been made to develop self-care and self-management programmes for children and young people (Department of Health 2007, 2009). The development of patient–professional relationships has been cited as one way of providing effective self-care support (Kirk *et al.* 2010) and therefore age-appropriate communication and engagement are vital. Evaluation of the evid-ence base for some self-care management programmes using text messaging and e-health interventions suggests they are effective methods of engagement for chil-dren and young people who have long-term conditions requiring self-care support (Kirk *et al.* 2010). An example of this can be drawn from a study undertaken by Franklin *et al.* (2006), whereby text messages were sent daily to young people with type 1 diabetes. These were designed to reinforce goals and information outlined in clinic. The study found that self-efficacy and self-reported adherence were improved due to the use of text messages.

Work recently undertaken by the Children and Young People's Health Out-comes Forum (2012) identified that young people want health service providers to use new technologies as a source of accurate and accessible health information. Older children and young people are more likely to engage in new technologies, a point that was recognized by Lord Darzi when reviewing the NHS as a whole prior to the biggest restructuring of the NHS since its inception over 60 years ago. Darzi (2008: 26) reported that new technologies provide 'unprecedented levels of control, personalization and connection' to children and young people. Utilizing new tech-nologies is seen as a positive strategy to engage and empower children and young people to take control and may support a therapeutic relationship where further health promotion can be identified. For example, a child or young person attached to their non-invasive ventilation machine overnight in the home may be required to begin their treatment at 6 p.m., meaning the bedtime routine starts very early. Public Health England (2013: 8) states 'wellbeing within families and family rela-tionships ... is associated with high levels of happiness and less worry in children'. Careful planning may allow a play activity that the child can do on their own to be provided, for example a computer game, or involving siblings and parents in a shared gaming platform within the home may prevent the child or young person from feeling isolated or singled out because of their health need. Similarly, older children or young people may be part of an online gaming community, thereby allowing them a degree of control and a connection that they otherwise may not have experienced.

Activity 7.4

- Can you think of other examples where new technologies have been used to engage children and young people?
- Can you think of any examples where the use of new technologies may not be appropriate?

The use of modern technologies such as the iPad and its huge range of apps can provide opportunities for play and recreation, as well as a tool for preparation and distraction. However, care must be taken to ensure appropriate usage policies and procedures are in place and are followed, as demonstrated through the case study in Chapter 8.

New technologies have been used by the Department of Health to target populations of older children and young people. An example of effective practice was recently highlighted through the campaign to encourage young women to have the HPV vaccine. This has been identified as one of the most successful public health campaigns in recent years, with a 60.4 per cent uptake for all three vaccinations for young women aged 12–19 years (Sheridan and White 2011). The campaign used peer role modelling, age-appropriate colloquial language and was targeted at the young women themselves. This shows how recognition and utilization of cultural contexts when promoting interventions for children and young people should be acknowledged and used (Open University 2011). Not only is this seen as good practice, but it also respects the person's fundamental rights (Gleave and Cole-Hamilton 2012). However, care must be taken not to patronize or assume adults know the best way in which this information can be provided. Kennedy (2010) suggested a lack of training may lead staff to treat young people inappropriately. This may be unintentional and provides another example whereby the perception of adults does not necessarily reflect the viewpoint of children or young people. This is demonstrated by work recently undertaken by the Children and Young People's Health Outcomes Forum (2012), showing that children and young people

- 'Want more information and advice about healthy lifestyles that is written and communicated in ways that resonate for them
- Want to be involved in the design, development and evaluation of child friendly campaigns and services
- Recognise there is a place for social media and want a trusted internet source of accurate health information.'

To support this, staff may need to undertake additional training to ensure they are competent and confident to engage and promote the use of these new technologies (Royal College of Nursing 2012).

Useful sources of further information

NCB Public Health event report (March 2011) *Healthy lives, healthy people: young people's views on being well and the future of public health*. This report provides a comprehensive overview of young people's perception in relation to health and wellbeing: www.ncb. org.uk/media/37997/vss_publichealth_report.pdf

Further reading

Baylliss Robbins, P. (2012) *Waterworld and treetops: designed* with *children* for *children: the new unit at Salisbury District Hospital*. 'A colourful insight into the process, teamwork, art and design that has created the new Children's Unit at Salisbury District Hospital.

Young Minds: 'At YoungMinds, we offer information to young people and children about mental health and emotional wellbeing': www.youngminds.org.uk/for_children_young_people

References

Aldiss, S., Horstman, M., O'Leary, C., Richardson, A. and Gibson, F. (2009) What is important to young children who have cancer while in hospital? *Children & Society*, 23(2): 85–98.

Allen, S. and Gordon, P. (2011) *How children learn 4: thinking on special educational needs and inclusion*, Leamington Spa: Practical Pre-School Books.

Baylliss Robbins, P. (2012) *Waterworld and treetops*, Salisbury: ArtCare Publications.

BBC News (2008) *Hospital roof-top play area opens*. Online. Available: http://news.bbc.co.uk/1/hi/england/leicestershire/7803577.stm (accessed 1 December 2013).

Bruce, T. (2011) *Learning through play: for babies, toddlers and young children*, 2nd edn, Oxon: Hodder Education.

Bruce, T. and Meggitt, C. (2005) *Child care and education*, 3rd edn, London: Hodder Arnold.

Carter, B. (2012) Children's well-being: priorities and considerations. *Journal of Child Health-care*, 16(2): 107–108.

CBBC Newsround (2009) *Adam checks out Wii physiotherapy for kids*. Online. Available: http://news.bbc.co.uk/cbbcnews/hi/newsid_7870000/newsid_7877800/7877879.stm (accessed 18 July 2013).

Children and Young People's Health Outcome Forum (2012) *Children and Young People's Health Outcome Forum: public health group factsheet*. Online. Available: www.gov.uk/government/uploads/system/uploads/attachment_data/file/198158/Public_Health_Group_Fact_Sheet_-_20130419.pdf (accessed 2 December 2013).

Children's Society (n.d.) *How to support your child's well-being*, The Children's Society.

Children's Society (2012) *The good childhood report 2012: a summary of our findings*, London: The Children's Society.

Cole-Hamilton, I. and Gleave, J. (2011) *Highlight no. 265: play and children's health and well-being*, London: National Children's Bureau.

CWDC (Children's Workforce Development Council) (2010) *The common core of skills and knowledge*, Leeds: Children's Workforce Development Council.

Darzi, A. (2008*) High quality care for all: NHS next stage review final report*, London: The Stationery Office.

Dawood, O.T., Izham, M., Ibrahim, M. and Palaian, S. (2010) Medication compliance among children. *World Journal of Pediatrics*, 6(3): 200–202.

Department of Health (2007) *Making every young person with diabetes matter*, London: Department of Health.

Department of Health (2009) *Healthy lives, brighter futures: the strategy for children and young people's health*, London: Department of Health.

Department of Health (2013) *Making mental health services more effective and accessible*, Online. Available: www.gov.uk/government/policies/making-mental-health-services-more-effective-and-accessible-2 (accessed 1 December 2013).

Department of Health – Children and Young People (2011) *You're welcome: quality criteria for young people friendly health services*, London: Department of Health.

Early Education (2012) *Development matters in the Early Years Foundation Stage (EYFS)*, London: Early Education.

Ewels, L. and Simnett, I. (2003) *Promoting health: a practical guide*, 5th edn, London: Baillière Tindall.

Fauth, B. (2008) *Young children's well-being: domains and contexts of development from birth to eight*, London: NCB Research Centre.

Franklin, V., Waller, A., Pagliari, C. and Greene, S. (2006) A randomized controlled trial of Sweet Talk, a text-messaging system to support young people with diabetes. *Diabetic Medicine* 23(12):1332–1338.

Gleave, J. and Cole-Hamilton, I. (2012) *'A world without play': a literature review*, Play England.

GOV.UK (2013a) *Physical activity guidelines for children and young people (5–18 years)*. Online. Available: www.gov.uk/government/uploads/system/uploads/attachment_data/file/213739/dh_128144.pdf (accessed 1 December 2013).

GOV.UK (2013b) *Creating a lasting legacy from the 2012 Olympic and Paralympic Games*. Online. Available: www.gov.uk/government/policies/creating-a-lasting-legacy-from-the-2012-olympic-and-paralympic-games (accessed 1 December 2013).

GOV.UK (2013c) *Public health: what we're doing*, Online. Available: www.gov.uk/government/topics/public-health (accessed 1 December 2013).

Her Majesty's Government and Department of Health (2011) *No health without mental health: a cross-government mental health outcomes strategy for people of all ages*, London: Department of Health.

Hospital Play Staff Education Trust (2013) *Play in hospital and the role of the hospital play specialist*. Online. Available: www.hpset.org.uk/role.html (accessed 2 December 2013).

Houlston, A., Buttery, E. and Powell, B. (2009) Cook to order: meeting the nutritional needs of children with cancer in hospital. *Paediatric Nursing*, 21(4): 25–27.

Hubbuck, C. (2009) *Play for sick children: play specialists in hospitals and beyond*, London: Jessica Kingsley Publishers Ltd.

Hutton, A. (2010) How adolescent patients use ward space. *Journal of Advanced Nursing*, 66 (8): 1802–1809.

International Network of Health Promoting Hospitals and Health Services (2012) *Children's rights in hospital and health services: assessment tool for health professionals*. Online. Available: www.hphnet.org/images/stories/Assessment_Tool_for_Health_Professionals.pdf (accessed 1 December 2013).

Jack, K. and Holt, M. (2008) Community profiling as part of a health needs assessment. *Nursing Standard*, 22(18): 51–56.

Kennedy, I. (2010) *Getting it right for children and young people: overcoming cultural barriers in the NHS so as to meet their needs*, London: Department of Health.

Kirk, S., Beatty, S., Callery, P., Milnes, L. and Pryjmachuk, S. (2010) *Evaluating self-care support for children and young people with long-term conditions*, Southampton: National Institute for Health Research Service Delivery and Organisation Programme.

La Valle, L. and Payne, L. (2012) *Listening to children's views on health provision: a rapid review of the evidence*, London: National Children's Bureau.

Naylor, C., Parsonage, M., McDaid, D., Knapp, M., Fossey, M. and Galea, A. (2012) *Long-term conditions and mental health: the cost of co-morbidities*, London: The King's Fund.

NHS Careers (2013) *Hospital play staff*. Online. Available: www.nhscareers.nhs.uk/explore-by-career/wider-healthcare-team/careers-in-the-wider-healthcare-team/corporate-services/hospital-play-staff (accessed 2 December 2013).

NHS Confederation (2012) *Children and young people's health in changing times*, London: NHS Confederation.

NHS Employers (2010) *Appraisals and KSF made simple: a practical guide*, London: NHS Employers.

Open University (2011) *Young people's wellbeing*. Online. Available: www.open.edu/open-learn/body-mind/health/children-and-young-people/young-peoples-wellbeing/content-section-0 (accessed 2 December 2013).

Oxford Brookes University (2013) *Wii Fit could help children with movement difficulties*. Online. Available: www.brookes.ac.uk/about-brookes/news/wii-fit-could-help-children-with-movement-difficulties (accessed 1 December 2013).

Philpott, J., Houghton, K. and Luke, A. (2010) Physical activity recommendations for children with specific chronic health conditions: juvenile idiopathic arthritis, hemophilia, asthma and cystic fibrosis. *Paediatrics & Child Health*, 15(4): 213–218.

Play England (2008) *Play and health: making the links*. Online. Available: www.playengland.org.uk/media/120486/play-and-health-policy-brief-03.pdf (accessed 1 December 2013).

Play England (2009) *Charter for Children's Play*, London: National Children's Bureau.

Play England (2013) *The wild network*. Online. Available: www.playengland.org.uk/our-work/campaigns/the-wild-network.aspx (accessed 1 December 2013).

Play Wales (2012) *Play: health and wellbeing*, Play Wales.

Playwork Principles Scrutiny Group, Cardiff (2005) *Playwork principles*. Online. Available: www.skillsactive.com/our-sectors/playwork/item/3298 (accessed 2 December 2013).

Pound, L. (2009) *How children learn 3: contemporary thinking and theorists*, London: Practical Pre-school Books.

Public Health England (2013) *How healthy behaviour supports children's wellbeing*, London: PHE Publications.

Royal College of Nursing (2011) *Healthcare service standards in caring for neonates, children and young people*, London: RCN.

Royal College of Nursing (2012) *Core competencies for nursing children and young people*, London: RCN.

Royal College of Paediatric and Child Health and NHS Confederation (2011) *Involving children and young people in health services*, London: NHS Confederation.

Royal National Institute of Blind People (2011) *Effective practice guide: planned play*. Online. Available: www.rnib.org.uk/professionals/Documents/plannedplay.doc (accessed 2 December 2013).

Scout Association (2012) *Rise to the challenge: exploring spiritual development in scouting*, London: The Scout Association.

Sheridan, A. and White, J. (2011) *Annual HPV vaccine coverage in England in 2009/2010*, London: Department of Health.

Skills Active (2013a) *Playwork principles*. Online. Available: www.skillsactive.com/our-sectors/playwork/item/3298 (accessed 2 December 2013).

Skills Active (2013b) *SkillsActive UK Play and Playwork Education and Skills Strategy: 2011–2016*. Online. Available: www.skillsactive.com/images/stories/PDF/Skillsactive_Playwork_Strategy_2011–2016.pdf (accessed 2 December 2013).

Skills Active (2013c) *The Pocket Guide to Playwork*. Online. Available: www.playboard.org/Uploads/document/290620110857-1455693788.pdf (accessed 1 December 2013).

Tylee, A., Haller, D., Graham, T., Churchill, R. and Sanci, L. (2007) Youth-friendly primary-care services: how are we doing and what more needs to be done? *The Lancet*, 369 (9572): 1565–1573.

Unicef United Kingdom (2013) *Report card 11: child well-being in rich countries: a comparative overview*, Florence: Unicef UK.

University College London Hospitals (2013) *About the Cancer Centre*. Online. Available: www.uclh.nhs.uk/OurServices/OurHospitals/UCH/CC/Pages/AbouttheCancerCentre.aspx (accessed 1 December 2013).

World Health Organization (2003a) *WHO definition of health*. Online. Available: www.who.int/about/definition/en/print.html (accessed 1 December 2013).

World Health Organization (2003b) *Adherence to long-term therapies: evidence for action*, Geneva: World Health Organization.

World Health Organization (2013) *Adolescent friendly health services*. Online. Available: www.who.int/maternal_child_adolescent/topics/adolescence/health_services/en/index.html (accessed 2 December 2013).

Young Minds (2013a) *Improving mental health*. Online. Available: www.youngminds.org.uk/for_children_young_people/better_mental_health (accessed 1 December 2013).

Young Minds (2013b) *What's the problem?* Online. Available: www.youngminds.org.uk/about/whats_the_problem (accessed 1 December 2013).

8

POLICY AND PRACTICE

Sandie Dinnen and Sue Ware

This chapter will discuss the utilization of policies and procedures within healthcare settings for enhancing the provision of safe and effective play and recreational opportunities for children and young people.

Chapter objectives

By the end of this chapter you will have an awareness of:

- the contextual background of policy development for children and young people;
- the relationship between policy and practice;
- the importance and relevance of policy for practice;
- how to use policy to influence effective practice;
- how to reflect on and evaluate policy implementation and assess its impact.

THE NHS KNOWLEDGE AND SKILLS FRAMEWORK

Quality
- Follows trust and professional policies and procedures and other quality approaches as required. Encourages others to do the same.

Equality and diversity
- Interprets equality, diversity and rights in accordance with legislation, policies, procedures and good practice
- Promotes equality and diversity in own area and ensures policies are adhered to

Service improvement
- Evaluate draft policies and strategies and feedback thoughts on impacts on users and the public
- Enables and encourages others to suggest change, challenge tradition and share good practice with other areas of the trust

(NHS Employers 2010)

THE COMMON CORE OF SKILLS AND KNOWLEDGE

Safeguarding and promoting the welfare of the child or young person

- Have the confidence to challenge the way you or others practise
- Have the confidence to actively represent the child or young person and his or her rights
- Understand the use that children and young people make of new technologies to understand the implications of risks of harm

Multi-agency and integrated working

- Understand that others may not have the same understanding of professional terms and may interpret abbreviations and acronyms differently
- Have the confidence to challenge situations by looking beyond your immediate role and asking considered questions. Be assertive about what is required to avoid or remedy poor outcomes for the child or young person.

(CWDC 2010)

Introduction

Policy is often considered the Marmite™ of professional practice. Practitioners tend to either love it or hate it. In trying to understand this attitude it is important to look at how policies are formed and what the drivers behind them are. Policy can emerge as a consequence of varying factors and the outcomes can be seen in many areas of practice today.

The development of new policies and procedures often emerges in response to incidents or events. The 'Cleveland Inquiry' (Butler-Sloss 1988) was undertaken following the removal of 121 children from their families, who had been diagnosed by paediatricians as the victims of sexual abuse by family members (Valios 2007). This removal of children from the family home was seen as detrimental to the child's wellbeing and subsequent legislation in the form of the *Children Act 1989* identified that wherever possible, children should remain with their families, unless intervention within the family was necessary (Department for Children, Schools and Families 2010).

Policy can also be in response to a tragic outcome that should have been avoided, such as the death of a child. The Victoria Climbié Inquiry (Laming 2003) followed by the publication of the government Green Paper *Every child matters* (Department for Education and Skills 2003) subsequently led to the *Children Act 2004* and a whole host of new policy initiatives and government-led strategies. Likewise, the publicity generated through the murder of Holly Wells and Jessica Chapman in Soham led to the Bichard Inquiry and one of the main recommendations was the need to establish a registration scheme for all people working with children and vulnerable adults, which could be accessed by employers (Bichard 2004).

All three of these examples, and many since, have identified that much of what had happened would have been avoidable if agencies had worked together more effectively, hence the continual drive for multi-agency working and the development of integrated services.

Policy development for children and young people

Politics itself can drive policy. A change of government or a new manifesto from a government in waiting to promote more people into employment can shape policy. If the government has an agenda that includes getting parents back into the work place, they will need to develop policies for good childcare provision to enable this to happen. For example, the government provides additional tax credits to help meet the cost of childcare places for working parents (GOV.UK 2013).

Research has been a major factor in influencing legislation, policy and best practice for those working with children and young people. Much of the research undertaken in the mid twentieth century has now become an established part of practice. This has informed both the educational and pastoral aspects of much of what we do today, and has been discussed in detail within earlier chapters of the book. The work of these pioneers continues today, with new theories being developed to support and challenge those that came earlier. These will no doubt influence the next generation of practitioners as they develop policies for the future. As an example, Play England (2013) are today promoting the role of outdoor play and engaging with nature, particularly in relation to children's health and well-being. This develops the earlier work of Frobel, who was a great advocate of the role of nature and outdoor play for young children (Pound 2005).

Looking back to some of the original thinking behind many current policies, it is worth exploring the historical context beyond the original research. In the case of attachment theory, the pioneering work is generally considered to have been undertaken by Bowlby, and later Ainsworth. However, work undertaken just after the Second World War by Freud and Dann (1951) focused on a group of six children whose parents had died in concentration camps and who were themselves severely damaged by the effects of war. They arrived in England and became the focus of a case study known as the 'Bulldog Bank study'. The study identified the importance of significant attachment figures in a child's life and noted that if the attachment figure is not an adult, then children can make strong attachments with their peers (Freud and Dann 1951). Thereafter, research undertaken by Bowlby and later Ainsworth greatly influenced the next generation of policy makers. From this research it is now taken for granted that children have a formal induction into early years provision which includes a more gradual separation from parents or carers with policies to support this and actively promote parental involvement in the setting after the settling-in period has passed (Early Education 2012).

Activity 8.1

When practitioners are inducted into the setting, one of the first things they are required to do is read the main policies within the setting and sign to say they will comply with the policy and its associated procedures. Think about when you last underwent a setting induction and the policies that you read.

- Were you aware of how the policy was developed?
- Did you think about why the policy and procedures were put in place?
- Could you trace the historical context of any of the policies you read?

In the health professions it was the continuing work of James and Joyce Robertson that had the most profound effect on separation anxiety for children in hospital (Lindon 2012). The Robertsons made two films on the impact of separation from parents linked to the changes associated with staying in a strange hospital environment. The evidence of obvious distress provided a clear indication that there were better ways of looking after the wellbeing of children who needed to be hospitalized. However, despite pressure exerted by James Robertson to try to change hospital practice, it was not until the films were shown on television that the medical profession, who had resisted change, were made to acknowledge the emotional and social needs of sick children. The influence of this work resulted in better policies and practices being adopted in the health community. This ensured an already traumatic experience was made less so through a change in the established culture of hospitals at that time. The innovative work of Bowlby and Robertson was decisive in changing conditions in hospital for young children, which is reflected today in unrestricted access for many parents visiting their sick children in the United Kingdom and other European countries (van der Horst and van der Veer 2009). This early work also led to the development of 'Mother Care for Children in Hospital' by a group of mothers in Battersea, South London, which became the charity Action for Sick Children (Lindon 2012), which has just celebrated over 50 years of active campaigning for child healthcare in the United Kingdom.

Activity 8.2

Within your setting, have a look at the visiting arrangements for patients who are staying on the wards. If possible, compare and contrast the following visiting arrangements:

- general wards for adults;
- paediatric wards for children;
- dedicated wards for young people.

The visiting hours will differ. Can you identify any policy or strategy documentation that supports the adoption of these visiting hours?

The activity above demonstrates that not all policy derives from legislation but can often be based on evidence to promote effective practice to ensure children and young people have the best support we can give them. Young people have been recognized as a distinct group who have defined needs which should be considered when designing, delivering and evaluating the services they use (National Youth Agency 2013). As a result, the Department of Health have published the 'You're Welcome' quality criteria for young-people-friendly services, which as a policy document, provides best-practice guidance for use at a local level (Department of Health – Children and Young People 2011).

Policy in practice within healthcare settings

For children and young people in hospital, best practice also includes ensuring that health and hygiene remain paramount in the daily work of those caring for them. Healthcare is provided within a wide variety of primary and community settings and 'healthcare associated infections' can be acquired by healthcare workers, patients and families that care for them (National Institute for Health and Care Excellence 2012). Controlling the risk of infection is vital and every hospital will have a policy that staff are expected to adhere to. Case Study 8.1 sets out why it is so important for healthcare professionals to be aware of the policy and understand how to implement it.

Case Study 8.1

The playroom has been open all day, offering a variety of toys and activities to cater for a wide age range of children and young people. Patients and siblings have open access and have been going in and out to play all day, often taking toys from the playroom back to cubicles or open bays. Around 4 p.m., when test results come through, a nurse comes to find the play specialist to inform them one of the patients' tests shows they have norovirus and the patient's siblings have been playing in the playroom. Norovirus is highly contagious and is known to be passed on via contact and on surfaces. The patient has touched some of the toys and it is highly likely the siblings of the patient are also carrying the virus, so the playroom and all toys the siblings have played with require a deep clean. As it is not always possible to know which toys have been played with and who else might be carrying the virus, all toys will need to be cleaned.

Norovirus can result in patients, visitors and staff becoming unwell with stomach bugs. Though this isn't generally serious to a healthy person, it can seriously compromise the health of a sick patient, depending on their condition. An outbreak of the virus can also result in the ward being closed to new admissions to prevent the spread of the virus, and in severe cases staff shortages, which is why good standards of hand washing and hygiene must be observed at all times to minimize the risk of spread of infection. Not only do these situations affect the wellbeing of patients, visitors and in some cases staff, but for play staff they can lead to a time consuming and potentially costly exercise that leaves other patients and visitors without access to the playroom and play resources.

The play staff's role is to empty the playroom so the cleaners can deep clean the room and furniture. All the toys need to be thoroughly cleaned, including those that have been taken out onto the ward. Cleaning staff may be willing to clean large toys such as trikes, but the majority of the cleaning will need to be carried out by play/ward staff. Any toys that are porous – such as books, puzzle pieces, unvarnished wooden toys, arts and crafts and so on – will need to be disposed of. Storage is often tight on wards, so many play resources are kept in playrooms on shelves or in open cupboards for easy access, so these toys will also need to be cleaned.

In these situations many trusts across the country have tried to limit play resources in an attempt to prevent the spread of infection. Policies and procedures can sometimes be blamed for restricting activities or the use of resources for no apparent reason. This is particularly true when considering health and safety while providing play and leisure activities for children and young people. However, limitations need to be carefully considered as excessive restrictions can seriously compromise the benefits and value of play.

Activity 8.3

Have you ever been prevented from undertaking a play or recreational activity or using a resource due to infection control measures?

- Why do you think the restrictions were put in place?
- Do you think the restrictions were justified?
- Can you think of alternative ways in which the activity or resource could have been presented or used in order to comply with the relevant policy or procedure?

The Health and Safety Executive (HSE), who support the provision of play across a range of differing environments for all children, has published guidance that aims to 'strike the right balance' to ensure the benefits of play are experienced to their full potential and uninspiring play environments can be avoided (HSE 2012). This guidance suggests that practitioners should use their own expertise as well as the judgements of others to make appropriate decisions that reflect the level of risk involved, ensuring any restrictions are actually proportional to that risk (HSE 2012).

There are sensible measures that need to be put in place to reduce the risk of cross-infection, which will enable time spent on cleaning and resulting costs to be minimized. These include:

- ensuring toys are purchased and provided following the Play Services health and safety policy;
- developing cleaning schedules so resources are cleaned regularly and maintenance of equipment checked;
- carrying out regular risk assessments over a three- to six-month period;
- keeping a departmental risk register, with actions reviewed monthly.

Receiving a thorough handover from medical staff can help to promote the control of infection. It is the medical staff's responsibility to inform play staff of any potential risks of cross-infection, but asking the right questions is essential. If informed a patient has an infection or is having tests, ask whether they or their visitors present a possible risk of spreading infection to others and whether they should be using the playroom. If this is the case then making up a toy box of activities that the patient and sibling have in the cubicle can help minimize the use of the playroom. Informing parents of outside play spaces for the siblings may also be helpful, while in some cases medical staff will ask families not to bring siblings to visit. These changes, which emerge as a result of practice, can then be embedded into the policy during subsequent reviews.

Knowing the play needs of patients helps with the setting up of the playroom. This way the play staff can ensure there are enough toys that cater for patients' and siblings' needs and remain welcoming but limit the amount of toys out in the playroom. Playrooms should be fitted with lockable cupboards rather than shelves and open cupboards. Not only does this help with potential cross-infection issues, but it means toys are securely locked away and out of harm's way when not in use. All toys that aren't being used should be placed in containers with lids, even those stored in cupboards, as this also prevents all toys needing to be cleaned if the cupboards have been left open or accessed. When putting out puzzle pieces and board games, keep them in plastic boxes with lids; this way the child or young person can still see the picture/game, but if they're not being played with the pieces are protected. The same applies when running activities as you only put out what is needed, keeping excess in a plastic box with a lid; this way not all the pieces will need to be disposed of in the event that this is necessary.

Cross-infection is also an important matter to consider when checking the design of any new cupboards or furniture. The safety, how resources will fit into the cupboards or how furniture will fit in the room tend to be the main areas considered and, though very important, cross-infection also needs to be kept in mind. For example, when new playrooms were recently fitted with very modern-looking and spacious cupboards, the doors had no locks and rather than door handles there were cut-outs in the doors that acted as door handles.

Reflection

Before the new cupboards could be used, what potential risks were identified and what action was taken to rectify the situation?

Play staff pointed out the potential risk of patients putting their hands through the cut-out handles to reach resources, the cut-out handles being used to prise doors open and the risk of infections being spread to toys in the cupboards. Play staff were asked to keep a record of any problems and report them via the trust's incident reporting system. The play team also decided to put these concerns on their risk register, which resulted in locks being put on the cupboard doors and play resources being stored in plastic boxes with lids. When the first cross-infection incident occurred, the infection control team informed the play staff they would need to clean all the toys in the cupboards as the cut-out handles presented a risk of infection being spread to all the items in the cupboards. As the play team had already identified this as a possible risk and kept toys in boxes with lids, play staff only had to wipe the boxes over. It also meant emptying the cupboard so the cleaner could wipe the shelves, and this was a quick and easy exercise. By risk-assessing the new playrooms the play staff identified possible risks and minimized them. This resulted in time being saved cleaning and sorting resources, cutting down on the cost of disposing of resources and, most importantly, protecting patients' and visitors' wellbeing while providing them with the important benefits of play.

The application of policy-related procedures

As demonstrated earlier, other policy may be in response to legislation, which will have been written to protect or promote the interests of vulnerable children and young people. The statute (in Great Britain the *Children Act 2004*) has been revised over a period of time, making it a dynamic and complex piece of legislation. It effectively sets the standards for a host of professionals working with children and young people; police, social services, health, education, youth work and more. Yet each of these different organizations will have different roles to play and this is where policy begins to make sense. Although we all have to adhere to the same standards, the processes for each sector and individual organizations within each sector may differ.

This breaking down of legislation into policies and procedures makes its application possible. For example, the role of the police when investigating a child protection issue is very different to that of someone working in health or education, whose role will be to promote awareness among children and young people of what they can do to safeguard themselves or how they will deal with disclosures in a professional manner. Therefore it is necessary for organizations to develop policies that are relevant to them, their staff and service users. A safeguarding policy in a hospital will clarify roles and responsibilities in supporting children and young people. A good policy will make clear the role of promoting understanding of safeguarding issues, the role of staff in handling disclosures and reporting procedures and, equally important, in keeping themselves safe.

Safeguarding policy and procedures need to be reviewed regularly and adapted to the changing needs of society. This is a very dynamic area where change is constant. With the advent of social media and an internet-based society there are more opportunities for children and young people to be exploited. The work of the Child Exploitation and Online Protection Centre (CEOP) not only investigates this form of crime, but provides some very useful guidance to children, young people, parents and professionals (CEOP 2013).

Activity 8.4

CEOP have developed a website called 'thinkuknow'. Using the following link, access this website and browse through the differing areas and resources: www.thinkuknow.co.uk

- How have they used differing design techniques to attract different users?
- How could you promote the use of this website for children and young people within your care?
- Do you think this should be your responsibility?

Case Study 8.2, taken from recent practice, clearly demonstrates the difficulties for healthcare professionals in balancing the risks children and young people should be taking as part of their development with the need to keep them safe and their need to understand the different policies and procedures within a setting and how one may interrelate with another.

Case Study 8.2

Incidents are part of everyday life and all healthcare professionals have a responsibility to safeguard patients, families and colleagues from potential risks and harm. The challenge for play specialists is that taking risks and learning from mistakes and accidents is how children and young people learn important life skills, so how do play specialists ensure they're not put off introducing potentially risky activities which benefit patients' normal development?

Though it can often feel like a paper exercise, carrying out risk assessments when introducing changes to the environment or new equipment is important.

This activity allows the play specialist to think through and problem solve any potential risks or hazards the new equipment or changes to the environment might bring.

No matter how thorough risk assessments are, incidents are part of life and they will happen. When they do it is important to follow the health and safety policies and procedures of the organization in which you work. However, following sets of procedures can result in patients' emotional or social needs being overlooked. It is therefore vital to be confident and aware of communication when dealing with incidents directly with patients. The following example of inappropriate material being viewed by a teenage patient via an electronic tablet will hopefully demonstrate how to investigate and report an incident balanced against meeting the patient's emotional needs.

Before introducing any equipment, a risk assessment to highlight any potential risks is required and trusts should have their own template of a risk assessment form which can be obtained via the health and safety team. Once risks are identified people are often tempted to overreact regarding what measures or actions are required to make a situation or activity safe. Sometimes a simple notice pointing out a potential risk is all that is required.

Electronic tablets offer a fantastic opportunity to introduce a wide range of resources as they are easy to keep clean and therefore accessible to all patients. Whether we agree or not, the internet for older children isn't just a means of looking up information, it's the way they communicate, stay in touch and function with the world around them. Coming into hospital can be an isolating experience for patients, especially older ones, taken away from friends, having their independence and privacy challenged and spending more time than they would normally like with parents and adults are just some of the frustrations voiced by many young people during a hospital admission. The internet overcomes many of these issues. It allows young people to stay in touch with friends, not only via email, but through the virtual world young people communicate in, via social networks and interactive video gaming sites. These sites offer the valuable opportunities for young people in hospital to stay engaged in activities with friends outside of the hospital and to continue to feel a part of their peer group, which is an important stage in teenagers developing their own identity, values and morals.

Unfortunately, the internet does come with risks, so when introducing electronic resources which offer internet access a comprehensive risk assessment is required. These are some of the questions that need to be asked as part of an initial risk assessment, to overcome many of the issues.

• Do you have the trust's agreement to provide internet access or are the applications (apps) on the tablets going to be used for entertainment and distraction purposes only? If so, how are you going to stop patients logging onto the internet?

- Are there the resources/personnel to maintain tablets?
- How will you prevent tablets being stolen?
- Is there lockable storage that can't be easily broken into?

When I introduced tablets to the play service I did so with particular thought to young people and improving communication between their peers inside and outside of hospital and therefore decided that internet access was required.

I asked our hospital school technicians for advice and negotiated having internet access via the school's website. Schools have a nationally recognized firewall so I knew this would be the play service's safest option.

Guidelines of use and terms of agreement formed with our trust's legal team were drawn up. Both staff and parents have to sign these forms to say they have read them and agree to take responsibility for ensuring the internet is used safely. Internet safety leaflets are also provided and discussed with patients and parents. It is important to take the time to introduce the rules and guidelines of use so that you can assess whether a parent has understood what responsibility they are signing for.

Next, a proposal with details of the aim of providing tablets with internet access, which included the risk assessment and action plan, was submitted to the trust's IT department, head of psychological services and child protection team for approval.

Once approval was received, tablets and lockable harnesses were purchased. A laptop also had to be purchased to enable the department to create an iTunes account so the tablets could be set up and apps downloaded. Restrictions were enabled on the tablets to prevent access to YouTube, the camera (preventing potential child protection issues) and deleting and downloading apps. Monthly maintenance schedules were drawn up to ensure restrictions stayed in place and software updates were uploaded regularly. Once all this was in place, a pack containing guidelines of use and staff and parent terms of agreement forms were given out to staff at a training session.

Incidents such as screens being broken and tablets stolen from playroom cupboards have occurred, but the most serious was an incident in which a teenage patient was able to access inappropriate material of a sexual nature via the internet. A student nurse shadowing the ward play specialists noticed the material the patient was viewing and reported it to the play specialist. The first thing that had to happen was to ensure no contact with unknown individuals had taken place and that the patient and other patients were safe from any potential child protection risks. The tablet had to be removed and handed to the school technicians to explore how the site had been accessed and measures put in place to prevent similar incidents happening again. The incident was then reported to the trust's health and safety team following the trust procedures. A discussion took place with the ward's social worker to explore whether there were any potential child protection issues and it was decided that the patient's parents should be informed in case such material is being viewed at home. The school also provided an internet safety lesson with the patient, play specialist and patient's parent.

While following these procedures, the play specialist also had to balance the feelings and needs of the patient involved, which is no easy task. The patient knew they were in the wrong so they denied it was them that had been looking at the site/material; this left the play specialist having to point out that they had been the only patient to use the tablet that day. The patient said it must have been left from the day before. Due to good professional practice the play specialist had followed the guidelines of use and checked the tablet at the end of the previous day, clearing the history and cookies. Therefore, because the play specialist had followed the guidelines of use it made it easier to be sure that it was the patient who had accessed the inappropriate site.

Remembering that teenagers are going to be exploring sex and sexuality due to their stages of development and the physical and psychological changes within themselves, lots of reassurance had to be given to the patient that the play specialist wasn't cross about the material they were viewing, and that it was the unsafe position they were putting themselves in that was the concern. This incident also offered the opportunity for the patient and play specialist to have a discussion about the patient's curiosity or any concerns they had regarding the material they had been viewing, which is why gentle handling of these situations is required. Having to manage incidents such as these can easily lead to bad feelings between the play specialist and patient, so the play specialist must sit back and think through how they are going to react if a situation like this arises. Serious thought needs to be given as to which other healthcare professionals need to know about the incident and if parents/carers need to be informed. If a patient feels everyone on the ward has been told they might feel humiliated and become untrusting of the play specialist, which can seriously damage the relationship and prevent the play specialist supporting the patient in other situations.

These situations need to be dealt with as a confidential matter and can greatly challenge the professionalism of play staff as they seek support in handling the situation. Mastering the handling of such situations really only comes through practice, but training and support is required so play staff can begin to understand how best to manage these types of incidents when they occur.

For the practitioner this case study raises many questions of how policy and procedures are shared and used within the setting. Without an in-depth understanding of what to do and who to discuss the various aspects with, it would not have been possible to provide internet access to young people who use this as a daily method of communication with their peers.

In dealing with the resulting issues sensitively and within the procedures of the setting, the practitioner was able to ensure that the resources remained available to other young people in the future, offering the potential for participation for a group who might otherwise feel isolated or excluded on a social level due to their hospitalization (Hagell 2012). The play specialist was also able to ensure that the young person involved understood the implications of his actions and was not embarrassed or humiliated.

Policy and procedures, like risk assessments, are often seen as paper exercises; however, if they are robust and written effectively they provide excellent guidance on how to deal with situations. They provide protection for staff and users alike and ensure that everyone is working to the same high standards. Baldock *et al.* (2007), writing on early years policy, identify the importance of consultation at government and local levels in developing policy. To ensure that modern policy meets the needs of the society it is aimed to inform, it needs to be forward looking, innovative and inclusive. It needs to be reviewed regularly and lessons learned from the past must inform the development of future policy (National Audit Office 2001).

What this means in real terms is that those working in a healthcare setting or any other organization serving the needs of children and young people need to consider themselves part of the policy-making process. If not directly involved in writing policy, they may be consulted and able to share ideas and opinions based on their own experience. They will be the people responsible for implementing the policies and procedures and will be the ones who can identify if they work in practice and are truly fit for purpose. It is the responsibility of the organization to ensure policies and procedures are in place and to inform staff of their existence, to train people to use these effectively and monitor them regularly to ensure they remain dynamic and relevant (Safe Network 2011).

There will be several policies and procedures in any setting; some will inform everyday practice, others will only be used occasionally. It is important that the practitioner understands how to access these and use them effectively at the right time.

Activity 8.5

Take time to consider which policies in your setting are designed to promote best practice.

- Who wrote these? Are staff, children, young people or parents involved in the process? How are these policies shared?
- Could this be improved in any way?
- Are there mechanisms for feeding back on policy? If not, how could they be developed?

The best policies and procedures will be written in a style and language that is accessible to all users. They will give clear guidance as to how they are to be implemented and will not be restrictive to practice, but will allow opportunities to promote best practice. They will take into account the culture of the organization and the users of that organization. They will be reviewed regularly to ensure they are fit for purpose and reflect not only current legislation but use proven and reliable research to support their development. They will be valued as one of the many resources available to those working with children, young people and their families.

Further reading

For a very simple but informative illustrated booklet on what Parliament is and how laws are made, download the Key Stage 2 resource *Parliament, laws and you* from www.parliament. uk Education Services: www.parliament.uk/education/teaching-resources-lesson-plans/ key-stage-2-booklet-about-parliament

The HSE have identified that people get confused by the difference between guidance, Approved Codes of Practice (ACoP) and regulations. This simple guide defines them and shows how they link to one another: *Health and safety regulation ... a short guide*: www. hse.gov.uk/pubns/hsc13.pdf

References

Baldock, P., Fitzgerald, J. and Kay, J. (2007) *Understanding early years policy*, London: Paul Chapman Publishing.

Bichard, M. (2004) *The Bichard Inquiry report*, Norwich: HMSO.

Butler-Sloss, E. (1988) *Report of the inquiry into child abuse in Cleveland 1987*, London: HMSO.

CEOP (Child Exploitation and Online Protection Centre) (2013) *Welcome to CEOP's thinkuknow website*. Online. Available: www.thinkuknow.co.uk (accessed 1 December 2013).

CWDC (Children's Workforce Development Council) (2010) *The common core of skills and knowledge*, Leeds: Children's Workforce Development Council.

Department for Children, Schools and Families (2010) *The Children Act 1989 guidance and regulations. Volume 2: care planning, placement and case review*, Nottingham: DCSF Publications.

Department for Education and Skills (2003) *Every Child Matters: presented to Parliament by the Chief Secretary to the Treasury by command of Her Majesty*, London: The Stationery Office.

Department of Health – Children and Young People (2011) *You're welcome: quality criteria for young people friendly health services*, London: Department of Health.

Early Education (2012) *Development matters in the Early Years Foundation Stage (EYFS)*, London: Early Education.

Freud, A. and Dann, S. (1951) An experiment in group upbringing, *Psychoanalytic Study of the Child*, 6: 127–168: reprinted in Freud, A. (1969) *Indications for child analysis, and other papers, 1945–1956*, London: Hogarth Press.

GOV.UK (2013) *Childcare and tax credits*. Online. Available: www.gov.uk/childcare-tax-credits (accessed 1 December 2013).

Hagell, A. (2012) Implications of new technology for adolescent health. *Every Child Update*, December 2012. Online. Available: www.youngpeopleshealth.org.uk/3/resources/18/ other-articles-briefings-blogs (accessed 1 December 2013).

HSE (2012) *Children's play and leisure: promoting a balanced approach.* Online. Available: www. hse.gov.uk/entertainment/childrens-play-july-2012.pdf (accessed 12 August 2013).

Laming, W. (2003) *The Victoria Climbié inquiry*, Norwich: HMSO.

Lindon, J. (2012) *Understanding child development: 0–8 years – linking theory and practice*, 3rd edn, Oxon: Hodder Education.

National Audit Office (2001) *Modern policy making: ensuring policies deliver value for money*, London: NAO.

National Institute for Health and Care Excellence (2012) *Infection: prevention and control of healthcare-associated infections in primary and community care.* Online. Available: http://guidance.nice.org.uk/CG139/NICEGuidance/pdf/English (accessed 1 December 2013).

National Youth Agency (2013) *You're welcome.* Online. Available: www.nya.org.uk/you-re-welcome (accessed 12 August 2013).

NHS Employers (2010) *Appraisals and KSF made simple: a practical guide*, London: NHS Employers.

Play England (2013) *Love outdoor play.* Online. Available: www.playengland.org.uk/our-work/campaigns/the-wild-network.aspx (accessed 1 December 2013).

Pound, L. (2005) *How children learn: from Montessori to Vygotsky – educational theories and approaches made easy*, Leamington Spa: Step Forward Publishing Ltd.

Safe Network (2011) *Help with writing child protection policies and procedures.* Online. Available: www.safenetwork.org.uk/resources/pages/writing_policies_and_procedures.aspx (accessed 1 December 2013).

Valios, N. (2007) *Progress in child protection since the Cleveland child abuse scandal.* Online. Available: www.communitycare.co.uk/articles/26/04/2007/104276/progess-in-child-protection-since-the-cleveland-child-abuse.htm (accessed 1 December 2013).

van der Horst, F. and van der Veer, R. (2009) Changing attitudes towards the care of children in hospital: a new assessment of the influence of the work of Bowlby and Robertson in the UK, 1940–1970. *Attachment and Human Development*, 11(2): 119–142.

9

INVESTIGATING PLAY AND RECREATION IN HEALTHCARE

Alison Tonkin and Norma Jun-Tai

This chapter explores how the effective provision of play and recreation activities and resources can be justified and enhanced through the use of investigative techniques and processes, together with the importance of sharing and disseminating your findings in a timely and effective manner.

Chapter objectives

By the end of this chapter you should have an understanding of:

- how to choose appropriate methods of gathering information within a healthcare setting;
- how to evaluate investigative techniques used to explore play and recreation activities and resources;
- how to use the information that has been gathered to inform the decision-making process;
- the importance of sharing investigation findings through dissemination.

THE NHS KNOWLEDGE AND SKILLS FRAMEWORK

Quality
- Works as required by relevant trust and professional policies and procedures
- Uses trust resources efficiently and effectively thinking of cost and environmental issues

Service improvement
- Evaluates own and others' work when needed
- Makes changes to improve service
- Passes on any good ideas to improve services to line manager or appropriate person
    - Staff feel they deliver a service to a standard they are personally pleased with

(NHS Employers 2010)

THE COMMON CORE OF SKILLS AND KNOWLEDGE

Child and young person development

- Know how to use theory and experience to reflect upon, think about and improve practice...

Multi-agency and integrated working

- Record, summarise and share information where appropriate, using information and communication technology skills where necessary
- Present facts and judgements objectively
- Be proactive, initiate necessary action and be able to put forward your judgements
- Know about tools, processes and procedures for multi-agency and integrated working, including those for assessment, consent and information sharing

(CWDC 2010)

Introduction

When promoting the use of play and recreation within a healthcare setting, knowing which resources or activities are the most effective in a particular situation comes with practice and experience. Knowledge about the child or young person's developmental levels is perhaps the most obvious consideration when offering appropriate play and recreation provision; however, other issues also need to be considered as 'attitudes towards children's play are socially, culturally and politically determined' (Open University 2010: 14).

This can be seen through recent policy statements from the current coalition government, who advocate the role of innovation and quality assurance processes, clearly promoting the gathering of evidence on which practice should be based:

> In a difficult financial environment, we need new approaches if we're going to improve quality and productivity. We think we can get more out of health and social care services if we encourage innovation and base more decisions on evidence about what works.
>
> *(GOV.UK 2013)*

The provision of play and recreation is enshrined in law and Article 31 of the United Nations Convention on the Rights of the Child (UNCRC) identifies the child's right to leisure and recreation (Unicef United Kingdom 2012). This is considered to be even more important for helping a child cope with illness through the use of play and creative activities while they are in hospital (European Association for Children in Hospital (EACH) 2013). Consequently, Article 7 of the EACH Charter states that:

Children shall have full opportunity for play, recreation and education suited to their age and condition and shall be in an environment designed, furnished, staffed and equipped to meet their needs.

(EACH 2013)

So how do you know what the right environment is, what equipment is needed or which staff will be able to meet the children's needs? Being able to clearly define what you do as part of your job role and how you do it is a fundamental element of practice. Tacit knowledge whereby an activity is undertaken or a particular resource is used but the rationale for its use cannot be articulated is not acceptable in the current financial climate when funding cuts have seen play specialist posts frozen and the downgrading of banding for some posts (Hospital Play Staff Education Trust (HPSET) 2013). The government, as stated above, want evidence of what works (GOV.UK 2013).

Working within healthcare settings means traditional research methodologies may not always be appropriate due to ethical considerations, particularly in relation to research governance within the NHS:

All research involving NHS patients, staff or resources must be assessed by a research ethics committee. Furthermore, to comply with the Department of Health's Research Governance Framework research activities must be formally approved by Trust management. ... Seeking Trust and Ethics Committee approval can be a relatively time consuming process regardless of the nature of the research proposed.... [However] many other activities are not research even though they use similar methodologies.

(NHS Research and Development Forum 2006)

Therefore, within this chapter, alternative investigation methods and activities will be discussed, starting from evaluation of your own role as a service provider through to evaluating services as part of a team or organization.

Investigation on a personal level through the process of reflection

Resources can be defined as 'a stock or supply of money, materials, staff, and other assets that can be drawn on by a person or organization in order to function effectively' (Oxford University Press 2013). This definition shows that a variety of factors need to be considered when evaluating play and recreation provision, and highlights the importance of resources for effective functioning of both the individual practitioner and the organization as a whole. Investigating these resources takes time, which is itself a valuable resource, so gathering evidence of effectiveness as part of routine, everyday practice should be undertaken wherever possible. This may be time consuming to begin with, but once established, it will become part of your routine provision as opposed to a separate, extra burden that appears to have little or no relevance to your practice. This has been demonstrated over the past 20 years in terms of the acceptance of investigating personal effectiveness through the process of reflection.

Investigative techniques and processes are grounded in theory which underpins the 'why' of our professional practice, making our role more visible to parents, children and multidisciplinary colleagues. This is dependent on an active engagement in reflective practice which enables practitioners to take a critical look at their work in order to inform future practice. Bloom's affective learning domain of receiving, responding, valuing and organizing future work (Curzon 2004) can be applied here and can empower the healthcare practitioner to take responsibility for not only how they learn, but also what they learn. Rogers argues that this 'increases curiosity, encourages responsibility and promotes personal and academic growth' (Petty 2009: 458).

Roffey-Barentsen and Malthouse (2009) highlight the work of John Dewey, a philosopher and educationalist who introduced the concept of reflective thinking. Dewey's theory can make us feel uncomfortable as we engage in the process of problem-solving a situation that challenges us, in an attempt to find a solution or new approach, but it is a powerful tool if it results in direct learning from the situation. Scales (2008) draws on Bruner's concept of the spiral curriculum, in which one area of learning can inform another by revisiting and building on ideas. Here, ideas and concepts are revisited over a period of time but at increasingly complex levels.

According to Roffey-Barentsen and Malthouse (2009), Kolb's four-stage model of learning recognizes that critical reflection based on experiences can generate new insights which include the processes of:

- Doing it,
- reflecting on it,
- reading up on it and
- planning the next stage.

This sits well with Schön's (1987) views on reflective practice whereby he identifies:

- 'reflection-in-action', which involves thinking about the action while doing it; and
- 'reflection-on-action', which involves the changes you make as a result.

Schön valued real-world learning and describes reflecting in practice as a situation occurs while simultaneously reflecting upon it, 'thus arriving at a considered response' (Gould 2009: 5).

McGregor and Cartwright (2011: 7) suggest that 'the aim of reflective practice is thus to support a shift from routine actions rooted in common sense thinking to reflective action emerging from professional thinking drawing from external evidence-based sources'. The application of Gibbs' reflective cycle demonstrates how higher-level reflective thinking links to reflective practice in order to demonstrate increased knowledge and skills in the workplace and the broader professional arena. Here, the practitioner can embed the cyclical process when they:

- Describe the event or situation,
- consider the feelings of the participant,
- evaluate the experience,
- analyse the experience,
- consider what could be done differently and
- take appropriate action.

(Gibbs 1988)

Activity 9.1

Consider your recent involvement in supporting a child or young person through an invasive procedure.
Can you apply the approach of Kolb, Schön or Gibbs to your actions?

Reflection tends to be done on an informal basis and unless an incident occurs which requires investigation through a 'critical incident analysis' or a practitioner needs evidence to support their own practice, reflection is seen as an individual process that mainly benefits the practitioner themselves. Another area that can be done on an individual basis but benefits the wider team of practitioners is reflection undertaken in a social situation, through the process of action research.

Action research

You may be prompted to investigate resources or activities as a result of recent training or as part of continuing professional development (CPD), clinical supervision or appraisal. Action research is another tool that enables you to use practice-based enquiry to identify and improve existing practice that is often part of progressive problem solving within teams.

> Action research is a term which refers to a practical way of looking at your own work to check that it is as you would like it to be. Because action research is done by you, the practitioner, it is often referred to as practice based research; and because it involves you thinking about and reflecting on your work, it can also be called a form of self-reflective practice.
>
> *(McNiff 2013)*

Callan and Reed (2011) advise that practitioners require knowledge, confidence and ability to investigate practice in order for the process to be 'bottom-up' rather than always 'top-down'.

> ### Activity 9.2
>
> Consider an area of professional practice which you would like to change and/ or develop.
>
> What is your driving force, i.e. why are you questioning an aspect of practice?
>
> Consider the impact of your inquiry – particularly on your colleagues.

The process of 'leading' change and developing practice is covered in more detail in Chapter 11, where the concept of leadership is explored.

Investigating individual resources or activities

This area is most closely aligned to the 'research process', and when undertaken formally it follows a similar pattern that should be identifiable through any research report or article presented in a journal or conference presentation (see Table 9.1 below).

A detailed discussion around the elements stated above is beyond the remit of this chapter. However, Marshall (2005) provides an overview of how to critique a research article, which could also provide guidance in terms of what needs to be included if you are writing an article yourself.

The Young Researcher Network (National Youth Agency 2010) provides an excellent toolkit that takes you through the process of undertaking a small-scale research project. This can be downloaded as a PDF document through the reference list at the end of this chapter.

One area that is often neglected within the investigation process – be it research, an audit or service evaluation – is the importance of undertaking background reading as it is often considered time consuming and not necessarily a productive use of time.

As an example of how important background reading can be, a poster entitled *Grab your gonads* promoting testicular self-examination will be explored.

TABLE 9.1 Standard presentation format for an investigation or research report

Introduction (what the report or article will cover)
Presentation of background reading (literature review)
Identification of how the resource or activity was investigated (methodology)
Presentation of what was found (results and findings)
Exploration and synthesis of the findings, including background reading, practice-based evidence and best practice (discussion)
Final thoughts having undertaken the investigation (conclusion)
What will be done as a result of conducting the investigation? (recommendations)

Activity 9.3

The poster can be accessed and downloaded for personal use at http://iheartguts.com/shop/index.php?main_page=product_info&cPath=0&products_id=214.

   Look at the poster and think about the design and use of the poster through the following questions:

- What is the aim of the poster?
- Who is the poster aimed at?
- What are the most noticeable design features of the poster?
- Where would you place the poster for maximum engagement?
- Why do you think this resource may be considered a 'play and recreation' resource?

Most of these questions can be answered intuitively; however, to maximize the impact of using such a poster, evidence needs to be gathered as it provides a context for undertaking the investigation and also places the investigation within the pre-existing literature (Lindsay 2007). The National Youth Agency (2010) suggests this stage of the process is simply finding out as much as possible about your area of interest, which in turn will help to define your investigation question.

   When originally undertaking the background reading for the poster, the following points emerged:

- men are reluctant to seek medical advice;
- men exhibit risk-taking behaviour;
- impact requires the use of humour;
- statistical information about the prevalence and age range of people affected by testicular cancer can be helpful to 'validate' the health message being presented;
- raising awareness of the link between early detection through self-examination and subsequent survival is necessary.

(Geoghegan 2009)

It was also identified that posters need high levels of exposure with the intended audience to be effective (Robertson 2008).

Activity 9.4

Look at the poster again and review your responses from Activity 9.3:

- Have any of your answers changed now you have a slightly more detailed knowledge about posters and men's health?
- Would you add anything to the poster? If yes, why? If no, why not?
- Where would you place this poster to ensure high levels of exposure with the intended audience?

Although this may not be an obvious area of involvement in terms of promoting play and recreation, the role of the health play specialist (HPS), as defined by the occupational standards, clearly state that 'the HPS should ensure that the environment includes health promotion resources' (National Association of Health Play Specialists 2013b). A growing number of settings now have dedicated areas for young people and these will often contain notice boards or areas where posters can be displayed. Therefore, not only will this resource promote health-related information, it does so in a manner that is considered to be the most effective in terms of design, siting and message content.

Having completed your review of the literature, you should now be in a much better position to go and investigate the poster itself, having identified the background information and the context in which posters can be used to convey health-related messages. This information will be needed again within the discussion section of the subsequent report, where synthesis of all the differing sources of information from the literature, best-practice standards and your practice-based findings are drawn together before finally leading to recommendations for changes that have emerged through the investigation process.

Moving from personal reflection and the evaluation of individual resources or activities to the evaluation of the service offered as a whole is far more complex and requires a very different skill set.

Why is it important for you to be able to evaluate the service that you offer?

Within the NHS, there is an expectation by patients that practitioners should be actively involved in the evaluation of the service they offer as part of the quality assurance process (Health Research Authority 2013a). This expectation is considered to be part of all practitioners' roles, although the level of involvement will be dependent upon your job role and level of practice.

Activity 9.5

If you work within the NHS, your job role will be positioned on the NHS Careers Framework at a particular level. Visit the following web page from NHS Careers and have a look at the differing job roles and how they are defined by professional titles, e.g. senior healthcare assistants at level 3 or practitioners at level 5. Locate the level you currently work at: www.nhscareers.nhs.uk/media/1695028/table-diagram.jpg

The overall heading within the NHS Career Framework descriptors that cover investigative processes used within this chapter is 'Research and Development'. Skills for Health (2008) define involvement in research and development across the levels as described in Table 9.2.

TABLE 9.2 Summary of research and development responsibilities across the NHS Career Framework

Level	Research and development
1	Contributes to simple audits or surveys relevant to own work area
2	Performs simple audits or surveys relevant to own work area
3	Performs simple audits or surveys and assist with occasional clinical trials or research projects
4	Assist with clinical trials or research own work area OR Evaluate equipment, techniques and procedures
5	Undertake straightforward or complex audit or assist with clinical trials or research projects
6	Carry out R&D as a major activity AND regularly undertake clinical trials or research projects
7	Initiate and develop R&D programmes
8	Implement R&D programmes OR Initiate and develop programmes with external impact
9	Takes overall responsibility for coordination of R&D programmes

Source: adapted from Skills for Health 2008.

The classification of investigative processes can be problematic and knowing whether an activity should be termed as research, audit or service evaluation can be confusing. This differentiation is important as research, as defined within the Research Governance Framework (Department of Health 2005), requires ethical approval by a Research Ethics Committee (REC). However, projects such as audits or service evaluation are not managed as research within the NHS and do not require REC approval or approval from NHS Research and Development offices, although organizational approval may still be necessary (Health Research Authority 2013b).

Activity 9.6

Having identified your current level of practice in Activity 9.5, look at the table above and identify what you should be doing as part of your job role in terms of research and development. List any activities you may have undertaken in the past, aligned to your level of practice, that demonstrate how you have undertaken this aspect of your job role over the past year.

The Health Research Authority (2013a) has produced a leaflet that defines the differing types of research and development activities that may be undertaken within the NHS. Access the *Defining research* leaflet via the following link and look at the table: www.hra.nhs.uk/documents/2013/09/defining-research.pdf.

According to the descriptions provided, would you define this activity as research, service evaluation or clinical audit?

As suggested in Table 9.2, formal research is considered to be a higher-level skill and it is unlikely that evaluation of play and recreation resources or activities will be formally researched as part of routine, everyday practice. However, with the current emphasis on improving quality and productivity, and the need for evidence of what works in practice (GOV.UK 2013), being able to evaluate the service you offer, through audit and service evaluation, is essential.

However, this is not a new concept; over ten years ago Belsey and Snell (2003: 1) made the following statement in relation to evidence-based medicine:

> Increasingly, purchasers are looking to the strength of scientific evidence on clinical practice and cost-effectiveness when allocating resources. They are using this information to encourage GPs and NHS trusts to adopt more clinically effective and cost-effective practices.

With the introduction of GP commissioning and the localization of funding away from central government following implementation of the *Health and Social Care Act 2012*, play services are increasingly being required to demonstrate their effectiveness and value for money, as demonstrated through the National Association of Health Play Specialists (NAHPS) conference in 2012, entitled 'It pays to play' (Hospital Play Staff Education Trust 2013).

Links to practice within a healthcare setting: clinical audits

Clinical audit is defined as:

> the process that helps ensure patients and service users receive the right treatment from the right person in the right way. It does this by measuring the care and services provided against evidence based standards and then narrowing the gap between existing practice and what is known to be best practice.
>
> *(Health Quality Improvement Partnership 2009)*

One of the first practitioners to realize the potential of data collection and how it could be used in relation to play services was Judy Walker at University College Hospital (UCH). Walker began gathering data on the use of preparation techniques for young children undergoing radiotherapy treatment. All children under the age of five years were routinely given sedation on a daily basis. Through the publication of evidence, Walker was able to demonstrate the effectiveness of play specialist utilization leading to employment of a dedicated play specialist in 2000 within the area. Subsequently it has been shown that:

> Children who have been prepared prior to treatment are less anxious, require less medication, demonstrate less maladaptive behaviour and cope better, which in turn can be cost effective for the hospital. Statistics show that within

two years of appointing an HPS for radiotherapy, the percentage of children aged between three and five years requiring general anaesthetic every day for a six week course of treatment decreased from 71% to just 22%. At an average cost of £18,500 per course, the financial implications are significant. Although factors are variable, the low general anaesthetic rates remain consistent at UCLH, with 11% of paediatric patients requiring general anaesthesia for treatment through 2008–2009.

(Tonkin et al. 2009: 13)

The benefits of this approach have also been documented by Scott *et al.* (2002) following a longitudinal audit over a five-year period in a regional radiotherapy centre in the northwest of England. An effective play preparation programme delivered to children aged 2–5 years had been used for many years, but its value had been implicit and unquantifiable. Through the use of simple auditing techniques, outcome data clearly identified a significant reduction in the need for sedation down to a level of approximately 10 per cent and no general anaesthesia (GA) for any child within this age range over the entire five-year period.

In 2006 the National Association of Hospital Play Staff commissioned Walker to write *Play for health: delivering and auditing quality in hospital play services* (Walker 2006) as a tool to evaluate and guide professional practice and development (National Association of Health Play Specialists 2013a). This is still the definitive guide for auditing play service delivery within healthcare settings. To complement this audit tool the NAHPS have recently developed a set of occupational standards to assist in standardizing and benchmarking good practice (National Association of Health Play Specialists 2013b).

Consider how the case study below incorporates the identification of the need to change practice and the use of auditing processes.

Case Study 9.1

More *et al.* (2008) report on the successful findings following the collaboration between a paediatric orthopaedic practitioner, hospital play specialist, consultant orthopaedic surgeon and a clinical audit manager. The aim of this project was to improve and standardize the care for children who need to have percutaneous Kirschner (K) wires removed. The study revealed the effective removal of K wires without a GA and reduced the time parents and children spent in hospital.

The procedure was effective for 90 per cent of children, but GA was necessary when the skin had sealed over the wires. This number could be further reduced if, at the insertion of the K wires, the wires left protruding through the skin are routinely bent through 90 degrees to facilitate removal. This study demonstrates how a cost-efficient service was developed utilizing the distraction skills of the HPS and the clinical skills of the orthopaedic practitioner.

Links to practice within a healthcare setting: service evaluation

Service evaluation is defined as:

> a way to define or measure current practice.... The results of the service evaluation help produce internal recommendations for improvements that are not intended to be generalised beyond the setting in which the evaluation took place. Service evaluation is designed to answer the question: what standard does this service achieve?
>
> *(NHS Direct 2013)*

Anecdotally, there is well-documented recognition that quality play services make a significant contribution to the way a paediatric patient and his/her family access and respond to healthcare plans. Following on from the work undertaken by Walker at UCH and Scott *et al.* in the northwest, involvement of play specialists is now seen as essential for good patient experiences when preparing children and young people for radiotherapy (Royal College of Radiologists *et al.* 2012).

Over time, this has been demonstrated mainly through qualitative evidence, although increasingly quantitative data is available, as demonstrated above. This mixed methodology should not detract from the message that service evaluation is possible using a combination of rich qualitative material and statistical data.

At a time of unprecedented NHS reforms and current austerity measures there is a growing concern that play and those who provide this service are seen as a 'soft' target due in part to a lack of awareness of the central and unique role of play in supporting the delivery of children and young people's health services. It is vital, therefore, that play service providers document, audit and evaluate their work in order to demonstrate the financial and psychological benefits based on intelligent service redesign. The need for this was demonstrated throughout Chapter 7 as 'All children and young people need to play. The impulse to play is innate. Play is a biological, psychological, a social necessity and is fundamental to the healthy development and well-being of individuals and communities' (Playwork Principles Scrutiny Group 2005).

The following case study demonstrates the steps taken by a play specialist to evaluate the services she offers using qualitative and quantitative data resulting in a cost-effective health service.

Case Study 9.2 is particularly important at a time when concern about children's dental health is growing, as thousands of children each year are having teeth extracted under GA due to dental caries (Manning 2013).

One of the key forms of data collection within service evaluation is the gathering of service user perceptions and experiences of the service offered. This increasingly involves the participation of children and young people themselves and this is covered in detail within Chapter 10. However, it is also important to note, that as participation of children and young people increases, the views of parents should also be considered. The *First Contact Care Survey* undertaken by Action for Sick

Case Study 9.2

Mimi Petty (2012) describes her work as an HPS in the operating theatre of a large university hospital; preparing, distracting and working with referred patients to minimize distress and maximize cooperation during dental procedures. Her initial enquiry into the number of children attending general theatres from April 2011 to March 2012 revealed that out of 1,973 patients, only three were unable to comply with induction through GA. These patients received further preparation from Petty and all but one went through with the procedure – the one remaining child was referred to psychological services.

Petty's work led to a permanent position in dental theatres and, following a period of clinical supervision, she was able to appreciate and address the specific needs of dental patients whose condition requires a GA compared to other medical and surgical conditions. Petty explains that parents may present with challenging behaviours that stem from their own anxieties, lack of ability and guilt at not being able to support their child's oral hygiene regime. Children and young people with special educational needs require an individualized approach in helping them to cope with physical sensations following a GA and loss of teeth, while understanding the temporary change in facial appearance.

As a result of auditing the number of patients requiring a GA, the cost of theatre time, cost of cancelled procedure and extended appointments due to anxiety and fear, Petty's role has extended to referral work to reduce the number of GAs as well as working alongside community dentists to promote good oral hygiene and diet.

Children (2013) surveyed 2,000 parents and the results were shared in the House of Commons in June 2013. The recommendations that emerged provided parents with a 'timely voice' with one of the most important outcomes being that health professionals need to provide reassurance at all levels and listen to parents as part of the contact process.

Sharing good practice

Having undertaken an investigation, audit or service evaluation, you will have generated information and evidence that needs to be shared. Lindsay (2007) suggests that this is the final part of the investigation process. Lindsay (2007: 92) goes on to state that 'dissemination isn't simply about making your research findings known, it's about making them known in the best possible way and about being prepared to defend them from criticism'. The National Youth Agency (2010: 21) concurs, stating 'you need to tell the right people about what you found out so that it can be used as evidence'.

Activity 9.7

Look back at Case Study 9.2 that described the work of Mimi Petty (2012) and the evidence generated through the service evaluation conducted between April 2011 and March 2012. Consider the following questions:

- How did the statistical data contribute to the establishment of a permanent position in theatres?
- What do you think was the motivating factor behind establishing this post?
- How has Petty's work led to the establishment of a sustainable and expanding play specialist post at a time when play service provision is being reduced?
- How did Petty disseminate her work?
- How would you disseminate the evidence generated? And to whom?

Lindsay (2007) identifies a variety of dissemination methods ranging across:

- submission of work undertaken as part of a qualification;
- writing a report and presenting this to your colleagues or managers (perhaps during a staff meeting or staff training);
- presenting a seminar paper to colleagues, members of the multidisciplinary team (MDT) or your managers;
- producing a poster presentation that can be displayed within the workplace (for example, during 'Play in Hospital' week, which is used to raise awareness of the role of play and recreation and the play services team within the setting for patients, their families and the wider healthcare setting community – see Chapter 11 for more details);
- presenting a poster or paper at a conference;
- publishing a paper in a professional or academic journal (such as Petty 2012).

Presenting at a conference, whether it is a poster presentation or an oral presentation through a concurrent session or a keynote speech, also provides the opportunity to network and extend the sharing process.

Suggested responses to activities

Activity 9.2

Sometimes colleagues may feel threatened when an area of practice is explored. Be wary of how they may perceive your inquiry through processes such as action research. Engaging your colleagues and getting them involved from the start, as well as providing a good rationale that explains the purpose and possible benefits of the research, may generate enthusiasm and active engagement as opposed to suspicion and negative feelings.

Activity 9.4

Possible additions:

- more detailed statistical information relating to the relevant age range
- contact details for more information or support

No additions:

- poster is generic and can be used anywhere – however, the above information could be provided in addition to the poster and contact information can be provided as tear-off strips for reference.

Placement of the poster:
To maximize exposure, the poster could be placed within a dedicated young person's room or clinic area or the male toilets. This website also provides similar posters promoting self-examination for skin cancer in English and Spanish and a poster explaining the menstrual cycle.

Useful sources of information

National Youth Agency: scroll through the website for a range of differing activities and resources for youth-led work, including some publications relating to research activities that are free to download via the publications tab. www.nya.org.uk.
I heart guts: provides a range of plush internal organs and other anatomy- and physiology-related products to help promote health-related messages, or prepare children: http://iheartguts.com.
Giant microbes: instead of plush organs, this site offers plush microbes representing a whole range of differing medical conditions and diseases: www.giantmicrobes.com/uk.

Further reading

Marshall, G. (2005) Critiquing a research article. *Radiography*, 11(1): 55–59.
Walker, J. (2006) *Play for health: delivering and auditing quality in hospital play services*, London: National Association of Hospital Play Staff.

References

Action for Sick Children (2013) *Action for Sick Children first contact care survey 2013*. Online. Available: http://actionforsickchildren.org.uk/action-sick-children-first-contact-care-survey-2013 (accessed 30 November 2013).
Belsey, J. and Snell, T. (2003) *What is evidence-based medicine?*, Hayward Medical Communications.

Callan, S. and Reed, M. (2011) *Work-based research in early years*, London: Sage.

Curzon, L.B. (2004) *Teaching in further education*, London: Continuum.

CWDC (Children's Workforce Development Council) (2010) *The common core of skills and knowledge*, Leeds: Children's Workforce Development Council.

Department of Health (2005) *Research governance framework for health and social care*, 2nd edn, London: Department of Health.

EACH (European Association for Children in Hospital) (2013) *The EACH Charter and the UN Convention on the Rights of the Child*. Online. Available: www.each-for-sick-children. org/each-charter/charter-and-un-convention.html#see-article-7-in-the-each-charter-click-here-to-view-now (accessed 28 November 2013).

Geoghegan, T. (2009) *Why are men reluctant to seek medical help?* Online. Available: http:// news.bbc.co.uk/1/hi/magazine/8154200.stm (accessed 30 November 2013).

Gibbs, G. (1988) *Learning by doing: a guide to teaching and learning methods*, Oxford: Further Educational Unit, Oxford Polytechnic.

Gould, J. (2009) *Learning theory and classroom practice in the lifelong learning sector*, Exeter: Learning Matters.

GOV.UK (2013) *Policy: increasing research and innovation in health and social care*. Online. Available: www.gov.uk/government/policies/increasing-research-and-innovation-in-health-and-social-care (accessed 28 November 2013).

Health and Safety Executive (HSE) (2012) *Children's play and leisure: promoting a balanced approach*, Health and Safety Executive.

Health Quality Improvement Partnership (HQIP) (2009) *What is clinical audit?* Online. Available: www.hqip.org.uk/assets/Images/Uploads/HQIP-What-is-Clinical-Audit-Nov-09.pdf (accessed 30 November 2013).

Health Research Authority (2013a) *Defining research: NRES guidance to help you decide if your project requires review by a Research Ethics Committee*, London: National Research Authority.

Health Research Authority (2013b) *Determine whether your study is research*. Online. Available: www.hra.nhs.uk/research-community/before-you-apply/determine-whether-your-study-is-research (accessed 30 November 2013).

Hospital Play Staff Education Trust (2013) *Hospital Play Staff Education Trust: annual report January 2012–January 2013*, Hospital Play Staff Education Trust.

Laming, W. (2003) *The Victoria Climbié Inquiry*, Norwich: HMSO.

Lindon, J. (2001) *Understanding children's play*, Cheltenham: Nelson Thornes Ltd.

Lindsay, B. (2007) *Understanding research and evidence-based practice (health and social care knowledge and skills)*, Exeter: Reflect Press Ltd.

Louis-Jacques, J. and Sample, C. (2011) Caring for teens with chronic illness: risky business? *Current Opinion in Pediatrics*, 23(4): 367–372.

McGregor, D. and Cartwright, L. (2011) *Developing reflective practice: a guide for beginning teachers*, Berkshire: Open University Press.

McNiff, J. (2013) *Action research for professional development*. Online. Available: www.jeanmcniff.com/ar-booklet.asp (accessed 30 November 2013).

Manning, S. (2013) *Stop the rot! Why thousands of British children are having their teeth taken out in hospital*. Online. Available: www.independent.co.uk/life-style/health-and-families/ health-news/stop-the-rot-why-thousands-of-british-children-are-having-their-teeth-taken-out-in-hospital-8527836.html (accessed 30 November 2013).

Marshall, G. (2005) Critiquing a research article. *Radiography*, 11(1): 55–59.

More, L.M., Proctor, I. and Henderson, A. (2008) The K Wire Project: removal of percutaneous kirschner wires from children without general anaesthetic. *Journal of Children's and Young People's Nursing*, 2(2): 66–76.

National Association of Health Play Specialists (2013a) *National Association of Hospital Play Staff milestones*. Online. Available: http://nahps.org.uk/index.php?page=history (accessed 30 November 2013).

National Association of Health Play Specialists (2013b) *National Association of Health Play Specialists occupational standards 2013*. Online. Available: www.nahps.org.uk (accessed 30 November 2013).

National Youth Agency (2010) *Young Researcher Network: toolkit*. Online. Available: http://nya.org.uk/dynamic_files/yrn/YRN%20Toolkit%20Dec%202010.pdf (accessed 30 November 2013).

NHS Direct (2013) *About research, service evaluation and clinical audit*. Online. Available: www.nhsdirect.nhs.uk/en/Commissioners2/WhatWeOffer/ResearchServiceEvaluationClinicalAudit/AboutResearchServiceEvaluationAndClinicalAudit (accessed 30 November 2013).

NHS Employers (2010) *Appraisals and KSF made simple: a practical guide*, London: NHS Employers.

NHS Research and Development Forum (2006) *Notes on developing procedures within NHS organisations for appropriate authorisation and management of research and related projects*, NHS Research and Development Forum.

Open University (2011) *The role of play in children's learning*. Online. Available: http://labspace.open.ac.uk/course/view.php?id=5653 (accessed 28 November 2013).

Oxford University Press (2013) *Definition of 'resource' in English*. Online. Available: http://oxforddictionaries.com/definition/english/resource?q=resources (accessed 22 December 2013).

Petty, G. (2009) *Teaching today: a practical guide*, Cheltenham: Nelson Thornes Ltd.

Petty, M. (2012) The cost effectiveness of the health play specialist role in theatres and the dental setting. *The Journal of the National Association of Health Play Specialists*, 51: 11–13.

Playwork Principles Scrutiny Group (2005) *The playwork principles*, Cardiff: Play Wales.

Robertson, R. (2008) *Using information to promote healthy behaviours*, London: Kings Fund.

Roffey-Barentsen, J. and Malthouse, R. (2009) *Reflective practice in the lifelong sector*, Exeter: Learning Matters.

Royal College of Radiologists, Society and College of Radiographers, Children's Cancer and Leukaemia Group (2012) *Good practice guide for paediatric radiotherapy*, London: The Royal College of Radiologists.

Scales, P. (2008) *Teaching in the lifelong learning sector*, London: Open University Press.

Schon, D. (1983) *The reflective practitioner: how professionals think in action*. London: Temple Smith.

Scott, L., Langton, F. and O'Donoghue, J. (2002) Minimising the use of sedation/anaesthesia in young children receiving radiotherapy through an effective play preparation programme. *European Journal of Oncology Nursing*, 6(1): 15–22.

Skills for Health (2008) *Career framework descriptors*, Skills for Health.

Turney, D. (2007) Practice. In: Robb, M. (ed.), *Youth in context: frameworks, settings and encounters*, Milton Keynes: Open University Press.

Tonkin, A., Alexander, A. and Mills, S. (2009) Let's play: part 1. *Synergy News*, November: 12–15.

Unicef United Kingdom (2012) *A better life for everyone: a summary of the UN Convention on the Rights of the Child*. Online. Available: www.unicef.org.uk/Documents/Publication-pdfs/betterlifeleaflet2012_press.pdf (accessed 28 November 2013).

Walker, J. (2006) *Play for health: delivering and auditing quality in hospital play services*, London: National Association of Hospital Play Staff.

10

INVOLVING CHILDREN AND YOUNG PEOPLE

Irene O'Donnell and Sharon Honey

This chapter will demonstrate how knowledge of children and young people's involvement in the planning, delivery and evaluation of healthcare provision can enhance the service being offered. It will explore how children and young people's participation can be incorporated into the health and care you provide and the benefits that this can bring for all involved.

Chapter objectives

By the end of this chapter you should have an understanding of:

- how to promote children and young people's own participation and involvement within healthcare settings;
- the benefits of participatory working for healthcare settings and the multidisciplinary team;
- the theoretical perspectives that underpin barriers to involving children and young people;
- the impact of patient-centred care on children and young people within healthcare settings.

THE NHS KNOWLEDGE AND SKILLS FRAMEWORK

Communication
- Develops partnerships and actively maintains them
  - Positive patient/public/partner and colleague relationships
  - Timely and accurate performance

Service improvement
- Enables and encourages others to suggest change, challenge tradition and share good practice with other areas of the trust
  - Staff adapt to change
  - Consistently improving care and service are provided

(NHS Employers 2010)

THE COMMON CORE OF SKILLS AND KNOWLEDGE

Effective communication and engagement with children, young people and families

- Consult the child or young person, and their parents or carers from the beginning of the process
- Make informed judgements about how to involve children, young people, parents and carers in decisions as far as is possible and appropriate. Take account of their views and what they want to see happen. Be honest about the weight of their opinions and wishes
- Know how to listen to people, make them feel valued and involved
- Understand the importance of building good relationships with children, young people, their parents and carers

Child and young person development

- Encourage children or young people to value their personal experiences and knowledge
- Understand that babies, children and young people see and experience the world in different ways

(CWDC 2010)

Introduction

Participation is a key word in current policy and practice. Over the past 15 years, there has been increased recognition of the importance of participatory working and the role that children and young people can play through giving their opinions and how this can contribute to making decisions and informed choices about their own health and care.

However, defining what 'participation' means in relation to children and young people is not easy.

Activity 10.1

Write down what you think participation means, then read through the following three quotations and make a note of the key words and roles for participation. Then try to write your own definition that reflects participation within your area of practice.

1   'The action of taking part in something' (Oxford Dictionaries 2013).
2   'The term is now used to describe many different relationships and degrees of participative activity. For children and young people this can range

> from them giving opinions on a particular issue (consulted and informed) to choosing their own agenda and taking their own decisions (child initiated and directed)' (North Port Talbot 2008).
>
> 3 'Participation is a process not an event and Empowerment is the outcome' (Crowley 2004).

These quotations all identify participation as key to taking part in something; however, the second quotation defines participatory roles and the third quotation identifies that the process of participation can lead to empowerment. Therefore, it is important that practitioners recognize that participation can mean different things to different people. For example, simply 'taking part' is not necessarily going to provide a positive outcome; consequently, to be able to develop participatory work everyone involved needs to be able to clearly define what participation is, what their role is, what they want to achieve and identify the resources and time needed to develop and support participatory work. This chapter will be exploring why involving children and young people is important by looking at current policy and government initiatives and their influences on current practice. It will also explore participatory approaches through theoretical perspectives and identify how these influences underpin participation and multidisciplinary team (MDT) working.

Why is it important to involve children and young people?

According to CommunityCare (2013), adults, children and young people cannot make a considered decision about the need for participation until they understand why participation should be integral to the workings of the organization. To be able to do this, an understanding of the legislative requirements of participation is required.

Participation is a right for children and young people and this should be reflected within policy, which is at the heart of service planning and delivery. This is advocated within Article 12 of the United Nations Convention on the Rights of the Child (UNCRC), which states that 'children have the right to participate in decision-making processes that may be relevant in their lives and to influence decisions taken in their regard – within the family, the school or the community' (Unicef 2013). The UNCRC was first introduced in 1989, and in the same year, the *Children Act 1989* put the child at the centre of this statute when the renowned phrase from this legislation stated that 'the welfare of the child is paramount' (legislation.gov.uk 2013).

However, it is really only in the last ten years that legislation has had a positive impact on participatory practice. In 2003, following the death of Victoria Climbié in 2000, the government published the consultation Green Paper *Every child matters* (Department for Education and Skills 2003), which identified five key outcomes that should be achieved on behalf of all children and young people. These stated that children and young people wanted:

- to be healthy;
- to stay safe;
- to enjoy and achieve;
- to make a positive contribution;
- to achieve economic wellbeing.

This was part of an extensive consultation process which identified failings across educational services, social services and health services. The *Children Act 2004* emerged as a result and this provided the legislative spine for the reform of children's services. This also gave further support to the need to listen to the child's voice. One of the main features of the *Children Act 2004* was the establishment of a Children's Commissioner for England to ensure that children and young people up to the age of 18 years, or 21 years if they are in care, can participate and have a say in decisions made about them (Office of the Children's Commissioner 2011). In 2005 another Green Paper *Youth matters* (Department for Education and Skills 2005) and the government's response *Youth matters: next steps* (Department for Education and Skills 2006) affirmed that the same five outcomes applied equally to young people:

> We believe that empowering young people gives a clear message that they are supported and trusted to make decisions. It gives them the chance to act responsibly and to assume an active role in decision-making and leadership in their communities.
>
> *(Department for Education and Skills 2006: 6)*

Next came the *Childcare Act 2006* which also highlighted the importance of listening to children and recognizing them as 'partners' in the planning and commissioning of services (Participation Works 2013a). With the introduction of the *Health and Social Care Act 2012*, two legal duties required clinical commissioning groups and commissioners in England to enable:

- patients and carers to participate in planning, managing and making decisions about their care and treatment through the services they commission;
- the effective participation of the public in the commissioning process itself, so that services reflect the needs of local people.

This includes capturing the voice of children and young people and this is reflected within the *Annual report of the chief medical officer 2012*, which devotes a whole chapter to 'the voices of children and young people' (Department of Health 2013a).

In order for participation to work, as well as meeting legislation, practice with children and young people needs to advocate a change of culture and attitude. Participation Works (2013b) state that 'A children's rights approach to participation reinforces the need for all those who are working with children and young people to ensure that participation happens as part of daily organizational practice and not just a one-off activity.' Participation must be seen to be a purposeful process where children and young people are listened to and actively involved in decision making, for if they feel unsafe and are not having their basic needs met their involvement in participatory practice will feel meaningless. At times adults will have to step in to protect children and young people regardless of their wishes, therefore involving children and young people in participation must be done in a way that empowers them. By regularly listening to children and young people, 'local partners can respond to children's needs, identify barriers to learning and development, and ultimately work towards improving services for young children and supporting children to achieve their potential' (Participation Works 2013a).

Theoretical perspectives

Historically children have often been vocal in protesting and criticizing the services provided for them in a local and wider capacity. Unfortunately their protests were often silenced by negative views within the media and/or physical punishment. The murder of two-year-old James Bulger by two ten-year-old boys in 1993 and the media coverage of the riots in England in the summer of 2011 have continued to reinforce 'moral panics' (Cohen 1972) about young people and their inappropriate behaviour. Locke (1632–1704) viewed children as 'empty vessels' and in this way babies were seen to be psychologically identical but thought to develop differently because they experienced life differently. Rousseau (1712–1778) argued that children are born essentially good and that poor behaviour reflects on a corrupt society. Both views suggest that adults are in control. This may be why, since the early twenty-first century, it has been a slow process for adults to accept the importance of encouraging children's participation. However these views have begun to change. By introducing participation alongside protection and provision, the UNCRC has acknowledged that those working with children must respect and value children in a safe, protected and participatory environment to build interdependent and empowering relationships. A positive impact of this has been the recent shift in viewing children as active, social participants, or 'social actors' (Prout 2005); no longer empty vessels, but young people in their own right who should be directly and/or indirectly involved regardless of their age, ability and needs within a range of diverse settings. This favourable shift in direction for children and young people has seen active attempts to capture views and opinions on their health and the services provided to meet their health needs. Several innovations include user groups, and patient feedback gathering is now an everyday occurrence in hospitals and healthcare settings. Gibson *et al.* (2006) undertook work with children and young people living with an oncology condition to explore their views on the services provided and transition from adolescent to adult services to help shape improvements. Projects like this helped validate the views and opinions of children and young people as being extremely important, given that they are the decision makers of tomorrow (Ansley-Green 2006).

Reflection

Think back to your own childhood and list the times when you felt you were involved in decisions that affected your life.

Draw a line across the paper and mark out a timeline from four years to 16 years of age. Now add significant events, such as when you started primary school, moved house, took exams. Think about how you felt when you experienced these life events.

Were you involved – do they feature on your list? If so, in what way were you involved? If not, how did this make you feel?

Sociologists such as Ulrich Beck and Anthony Giddens argue that contemporary Western cultures have entered a period of late modernity where Western societies are being shaped by a process of individualization (Beck 1992). Here, the relationship between the individual and the society are also influenced by new economic and technological processes. The experience of being active meaning makers by taking part in ordinary routines and practices on individuals enables them to make sense of their world and their place within it.

Beck (1992) characterizes individualization through three key aspects:

1 Disembedding – 'liberating dimension' – removal from familial and traditional ties.
2 Loss of traditional security – 'disenchantment dimension'.
3 Re-embedding – 'reintegration dimension' – creation of a new type of social commitment.

Activity 10.2

Try to complete Table 10.1, thinking about 'individualization and going into hospital' and the impact this may have on the child or young person. The first example has been given within each dimension.

TABLE 10.1 Complete the table with further examples

Disembedding – liberating	*Loss of security – disenchantment*	*Re-embedding – reintegration*
Having to leave home	Loss of guidance, practical knowledge	New social practices
	Religious faith	

Note: Did you consider the impact on the adults as well?

Identifying the importance of a practitioner's own biography and their 'reflexive project of self' (Giddens 1992) on practice is vital in understanding how personal experiences, personal values and skills can impact on a practitioner's practice with young people. By understanding the self, a practitioner is more likely to relate to a young person by reflecting on a similar experience/situation through their own choice biographies (Beck 1992) and their own identity – for example, gender, age, race and culture. This can in turn provide a broader understanding of young people and the meaning of practice, which can lead to empowering both the young person and practitioner. This supports the biographical perspective of recognizing the importance of how young people relate to adults and each other to negotiate their own biographical discourse. Identity is not fixed and continues to change, enabling the practitioner and young person to reflect on who they are and who they want to be. However, it is important to challenge Giddens' (1992) 'reflexive project of self' and Beck's (1992) choice biography approach for being too simplistic, as not every individual is able to control their own experiences, decisions and biographical pathway. Practitioners are often constrained by shifts within power between politics, the field they work in and the relationship between practice and theory.

Activity 10.3

Reflect back on the timeline you completed earlier. Were you able to make your own biographical choices? Were your experiences and decisions influenced by the reflexive project of self?

Is a terminally ill child or young person able to make their own biographical choices?

A child or young person who is emotionally intelligent is more able to accept and cope with a traumatic experience through recognizing their own feelings and the feelings of others.

The practitioner's ability to reflect on their personal skills, values, knowledge and practice is vital in how they improve practice and thus benefit the young people. Schön (1983) identified two processes: *reflection-on-action*, in which the practitioner reflects on what they have done, how it went and what could be done differently; and *reflection-in-action*, in which the practitioners use their knowledge from previous experiences and then apply this to make links between theory and practice (see Chapter 9).

When working with children and young people in healthcare settings it is important that the practitioner takes into consideration the whole picture of the child and how their family, community, culture and societal interactions have helped to develop the child's sense of self.

Involving children and young people: examples of participation in practice

According to Article 1 of the UNCRC, a child is defined as any human being below the age of 18 years (Unicef United Kingdom 2013). It is now generally recognized that adolescence is a separate developmental transition between childhood and adulthood with a different set of needs to that of a child. Adolescence can be defined as the beginning at puberty (12–13 years) and finishing at 18 years (Department of Health – Children and Young People 2011). With this in mind the government has acknowledged that young people are a distinct group within health services, and published '*You're welcome*', which identified a set of quality criteria that describe how healthcare can be made 'young people friendly' (Department of Health – Children and Young People 2011). The '*You're Welcome*' quality criteria outline a set of ten standards that were established to support health providers implement Standard Four of the National Service Framework for children, young people and maternity services (NSF) (National Youth Agency 2013). One of the most refreshing findings of the NSF policy was that children are not mini adults and should not be treated as such (Department of Health 2003). This led to the quality criteria being published to further publicize the needs of this patient group.

For most general hospitals, getting the environment right can be a challenge as young people tend to be cared for on either a paediatric ward or an adult ward. From work carried out with young people's focus groups it is clear that this is something they struggle with. Many felt uncomfortable sharing a ward with young children, but equally with older people too, and this can affect their emotional wellbeing (NHS Estates 2004). Therefore it is vital to make the space and opportunity for young people to be cared for in age-appropriate settings with activity and socialization opportunities available to them (Department of Health – Children and Young People 2011). If these facilities are not provided it can have a negative impact on how young people engage with their healthcare and treatment and effects can be both physical and psychological.

The charity Action for Sick Children (2013) has been at the forefront for many years of striving to ensure that health services for children and young people are of the highest standard and fit for purpose. Action for Sick Children (Scotland) is a member of the European Association for Children in Hospital (EACH) and in the EACH Charter they call for all staff caring for children to be specifically trained to understand and respond to their clinical, emotional, developmental and cultural needs (EACH 2013). For children and young people with chronic health conditions this is vital if we hope to minimize the impacts their health has on other aspects of their lives.

Hospitalization and the treatments involved can vary in the impact on children and young people, depending on their age, development, level of cognition and coping abilities. For younger children these can manifest as feelings of frustration, fear and confusion. For young people issues can include body image, self-esteem and compliance with medical treatment and regimes. Some children will be born with pre-existing conditions and live and grow with them as part of who they are, never knowing any difference. Others will have to learn to adjust to a diagnosis and the changes to their life for them and their family, and thus impacts experienced can differ significantly.

Health and wellbeing in the early years of life have a huge impact on health into adulthood and shapes how adults engage with healthcare (Department of Health 2013b). Due to this the delivery of quality care which provides positive experiences is crucial through birth to the teenage years to enable children with chronic health conditions to transition smoothly into adult services (Kennedy 2010). Children and adolescents going into hospital will always need support from those around them and they may have questions and anxieties they need to discuss (Action for Sick Children (Scotland) n.d.). As children enter adolescence, the questions they may have felt comfortable discussing with their parents may now seem too private or embarrassing and so it commonly falls to healthcare professionals, particularly play specialists, to take on this role as a trusted adult (White *et al.* 2006). Healthcare professionals working with children act as advocates for their patients and become trusted carers for children with long-term conditions, seeing them grow up, learn to take responsibility for their own health and move on to adult services. Enabling young people to actively participate in their healthcare supports those living with a long-term illness to gain a sense of control and responsibility in their life, which is often something they lose out on from having to live with a condition. Young people living with chronic illness face unique challenges in accomplishing the developmental tasks of adolescence (Louis-Jacques and Sample 2011). Risk taking is normal adolescent behaviour but there is some evidence to support the theory that chronic illness effects normal psycho-social development (Louis-Jacques and Sample 2011).

The United Kingdom still lags behind its European counterparts when it comes to health outcomes for children, but now at least it encourages its young patients to have a say in their healthcare. This should enhance a child's or young person's experience of healthcare and go some way to helping healthcare professionals understand more fully the impacts of illness for children and young people. Service providers should look at the way transition services are delivered for young people. Recently the concepts of collaborating on delivery and design of services have been successful models of engaging young people to manage their long-term conditions such as diabetes (Royal College of Nursing 2013). The recent Royal College of Nursing (2013) publication *Lost in transition: moving young people between child and adult health services* outlines a series of recommendations which includes involving young people in the design of services that are offered to them, letting them take an active role and showing that their recommendations are acted upon. Good engagement in the transition period can result in fewer missed appointments, greater compliance and young people being more informed regarding their own health (Royal College of Nursing 2013). Local health systems need to have govern-ance and policies in place to ensure children and young people can participate in a systematic and non-tokenistic way. This links in with the government's aims to increase participation with the 'No decisions about me without me' policy (Department of Health 2012). It is important that children and young people understand why they are being consulted, what the process is, how their feedback will be used and, crucially, how their involvement will lead to change or help professionals. Children and young people need to be engaged early in the design of new health organizations and structures to ensure their views are included right from the start and regularly in the future.

Case Study 10.1

University College London Hospitals (UCLH) NHS Foundation Trust is a leader in the care of children and young people. To reflect this we have recently developed and designed an innovative and interactive website for patients (UCLH 2011). The National Children's Bureau (NCB) has championed the meaningful involvement and participation of children and young people in matters affecting their lives, including health.

The website provides children and young patients with an opportunity to explore and familiarize themselves with a ward or hospital environment by watching films. It introduces them to some of the people they will meet before they attend the hospital. Providing age-appropriate information in different ways was an important aspect within the design. The Kennedy Review (2010) highlighted this as vital for children and young people accessing healthcare. By informing our patients of what to expect and what to bring with them when they come to UCLH we aim to reduce any anxiety or uncertainty. It also ensures that we are being efficient with our time and resources.

Based on a model of participation by Treseder (1997) the project was designed to ensure shared decision making took place. Patients and families were involved throughout the website design process. It is well documented that patient participation is integral to help shape services around users. We worked with a youth-specific digital agency specializing in creating content for and with young people in the United Kingdom. The following were used to engage our patients: focus groups, mood boards, design workshops using illustrators and graphic designers.

Developing the new website with patients for our patients has been an opportunity to engage in a rewarding joint patient and staff project. This has led to regular and continued patient participation on everyday issues such as food and visiting times and larger projects such as improving the environment, which we are currently involving our patients in as part of the planning and redesign of our wards.

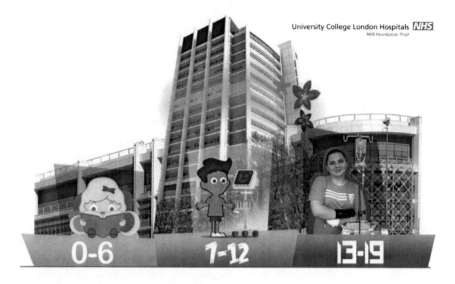

FIGURE 10.1 University College London Hospitals (reproduced by kind permission UCLH 2013).

Activity 10.4

Does your trust have a dedicated area for children and young people on their website?

Look at the UCLH site or look for a children's and young people's website in another setting.

- What is included on the website?
- How do patients get told about the website?
- Is it used for preparation prior to hospital visits, admission and procedures?

Why is it important that children and young people see peer presentations of information about health-related procedures?

Young Children's Voices Network: National Children's Bureau

Participation with older children has been well established, but there is less involvement with younger children – who still have the right to participate in their health and have a say on what they feel or need. Children have distinctive views and information to offer as only they know how they feel and what is important to them. Listening provides opportunities for young children to learn that their views about their daily lives are valued. NCB introduced a project to help lead participation with younger children, called the Young Children's Voices Network. For the project listening champions were introduced, comprising practitioners who have received training in listening, were part of a listening network and were dedicated to ensuring their settings were listening to young children and enabling participation. Listening champions promoted the importance of listening and supporting staff in developing and embedding listening cultures. A good example of this in action is displaying children's perspectives in the setting as it provides feedback to young children that their views are listened to and valued. Involve young children as much as possible in how their perspectives are shown, including their interpretations and their decisions about what is important (Young Children's Voices Network 2009).

To gather feedback from younger children, creative thinking is being used by some hospital trusts to engage with this patient group. Basildon and Thurrock University Hospitals (2013) have used a washing line of 'Tell us what is tops and pants about your visit' so young children write or draw onto a 'top' (positive) or 'pants' (negative) to give their feedback.

As discussed in Chapter 11, ideas like this can also be shared through social media sites such as Twitter: 'here's our washing line of feedback … [link to picture which is shown as part of the tweet] no pants there!' (Evans 2013).

At UCLH NHS Foundation Trust, a postcard feedback system was introduced whereby the play specialist would give each patient on the ward a postcard to write or draw:

1   things that you liked
2   things we could do better.

A bird box post box was provided in the reception area where the young patients could get their postcards stamped by the receptionist before posting. The information is collated each month and one good thing and one thing for improving the service are chosen to display and show how the issues are being addressed.

Every two years Young NCB members choose subjects that they think are the big issues for children and young people. They then find ways of addressing these issues through talking to the government, hosting events or doing activities that will increase awareness of these issues with other children and young people, adults and decision makers. The NCB and Council for Disabled Children have produced a new film, *Talking health*, which looks at what is important to children and young people about their health. The film was made with support from other organizations, including Young NCB and the Race Equality Foundation. Children had the chance to share their thoughts and opinions with growing confidence after taking part in activities that helped form their ideas (NCB 2013). Christine Lenehan, co-chair of the Children and Young People's Health Outcomes Forum and Director of the Council for Disabled Children stated that 'Talking health is a key tool which shows children and young people's understanding of health and what it means to them, it shows that not only do children have a voice but that what they have to say is valuable' (NCB 2013).

Working with the multidisciplinary team

Government policy and the legislative frameworks along with societal and media portrayal can influence, restrain and define the actions of practitioners. The Laming Report (Laming 2003) following the death of Victoria Climbié introduced a restructuring of multi-agencies to ensure communication and needs of the child and families were paramount, as defined within the *Children Act 2004*. A positive impact was the introduction of more MDTs working together to form various strategic partnerships and actions across voluntary, private and statutory sectors.

'Practice involves the purposive use of knowledge, and this incorporates two different (but connected) elements: knowledge *about* (that is, content knowledge) and knowledge *how to* (that is, skills based, process knowledge)' (Turney 2007: 57). Therefore practitioners need to not only reflect on what they know, their practice and what could be improved, but analyse this knowledge and question discourses by comparing work with other professionals, to develop the practitioner's and young person's relationship, empowering and giving autonomy to all involved.

It is clear from the discussion and evidence that exists that involving children and young people in their healthcare and decision-making process is a positive thing that reaps many benefits for the children and the organization (Royal College of Paediatrics and Child Health 2012). There is a need to extend the evidence base for the psycho-social wellbeing of chronically ill children, young people and their siblings in the United Kingdom to further support their transition into adult services. Advances in medical science have increased the number of children living longer with chronic illness with a consequent change in the requirement and demand for more and different services. Better understanding of the needs of this group is likely to lead to an increased ability to meet their needs holistically using knowledge and understanding of the support they require. Children and young people are key stakeholders in the health service and not just beneficiaries or passive recipients of services. Meaningful participation of children and young people in all aspects of the health system is important if health services are to remain relevant, high quality and holistic, and empower children and young people to feel valued. Long term, the hope would be that this will lead to an increase in the holistic wellbeing of children and young people using the health service; and better outcomes equals better lives.

Further reading

Annual report of the chief medical officer 2012.

Children and participation: research, monitoring and evaluation with children and young people: www.savethechildren.org.uk/resources/online-library/children-and-participation-research-monitoring-and-evaluation-children-and.

Children's participation (short open-access course from the Open University): www.open.edu/openlearn/body-mind/health/children-and-young-people/childrens-participation/content-section-0.

Involving children and young people in healthcare: a planning tool. Action for Sick Children and the NHS National Centre for Involvement.

Let's listen: young children's voices – profiling and planning to enable their participation in children's services: www.ncb.org.uk/media/71974/let_slisten.pdf.

Listening to children's views on health provision: a rapid review of the evidence: www.ncb.org.uk/what-we-do/research/research-projects/a-z-research-projects/listening-to-children%E2%80%99s-views-on-health-provision-%E2%80%93-a-rapid-review-of-the-evidence.

Weil, L. (2013) *Chapter 4: The voices of children and young people*: www.gov.uk/government/uploads/system/uploads/attachment_data/file/252654/33571_2901304_CMO_Chapter_4.pdf

Young Minds (2013) *Youth Engagement*: www.youngminds.org.uk/training_services/youthengagement.

References

Action for Sick Children (2013) *Welcome to Action for Sick Children*. Online. Available: http://actionforsickchildren.org.uk (accessed 11 December 2013).

Action for Sick Children (Scotland) (n.d.) *Young people in hospital*, Edinburgh: Action for Sick Children.

Ansley-Green, A. (2006) *The work of the Children's Commissioners*. Online. Available: www.publications.parliament.uk/pa/jt200506/jtselect/jtrights/uc1672-i/uc167202.htm (accessed 11 December 2013).

Basildon and Thurrock University Hospitals (2013) *Smile and the hospital ward smiles with you*. Online. Available: www.basildonandthurrock.nhs.uk/index.php?option=com_content&view=article&id=542:smile-and-the-hospital-ward-smiles-with-you&catid=9:press-releases&Itemid=212 (accessed 11 December 2013).

Beck, U. (1992) *Risk society: towards a new modernity*, London: Sage Publications.

Cohen, S. (1972) *Folk devils and moral panics*, London: Paladin.

CommunityCare (2013) *Proven practice: involving children and young people in decision-making*. Online. Available: www.communitycare.co.uk/articles/22/05/2009/111629/proven-practice-involving-children-and-young-people-in-decision-making.htm (accessed 10 December 2013).

Crowley, A. (2004) *Children and young people's participation: working towards a definition*. Online. Available: www.participationworkerswales.org.uk/participation-in-wales.aspx (accessed 30 July 2013).

CWDC (Children's Workforce Development Council) (2010) *The common core of skills and knowledge*, Leeds: Children's Workforce Development Council.

Department for Education and Skills (DfES) (2003) *Every child matters*, London: DfES.

Department for Education and Skills (DfES) (2005) *Youth matters*, London: DfES.

Department for Education and Skills (DfES) (2006) *Youth matters: next steps*, London: DfES.

Department of Health (2003) *Getting the right start: national service framework for children standard for hospital services*, London: Department of Health.

Department of Health (2012) *Liberating the NHS: no decision about me, without me – government response to the consultation*, London: Department for Education.

Department of Health (2103a) *Annual report of the chief medical officer 2012: our children deserve better – prevention pays*. Online. Available: www.gov.uk/government/publications/chief-medical-officers-annual-report-2012-our-children-deserve-better-prevention-pays (accessed 10 December 2013).

Department of Health (2013b) *Giving all children a healthy start in life*. Online. Available: www.gov.uk/government/policies/giving-all-children-a-healthy-start-in-life (accessed 11 December 2013).

Department of Health – Children and Young People (2011) *You're welcome: quality criteria for young people friendly health services*, London: Department of Health.

EACH (European Association for Children in Hospital) (2013) *The EACH Charter*. Online. Available: www.each-for-sick-children.org/each-charter.html (accessed 11 December 2013).

Evans, K. (2013) *Rt '@jerushaMK: @cazdilks here's our washing line of feedback #smilevember pic. twitter.com/XFjY1DVwMD' no pants there! @nahpsofficial @ACCNUK* (Twitter), 16 November. Online. Available: https://twitter.com/kathevans2/status/4016402 75036356608 (accessed 12 December 2103).

Gibson, F., Edwards, J., Sepion, B. and Richardson, A. (2006) Cancer-related fatigue in children and young people: survey of healthcare professionals' knowledge and attitudes. *European Journal of Oncology Nursing*, 10(4): 311–316.

Giddens, A. (1992) *The transformation of intimacy: sexuality, love and eroticism in modern societies*, Stanford, CA: Stanford University Press.

Kennedy, I. (2010) *Getting it right for children and young people: overcoming cultural barriers in the NHS so as to meet their needs*, London: Department of Health.

Legislation.gov.uk (2013) *Children Act 1989*. Online. Available: www.legislation.gov.uk/ ukpga/1989/41/section/1 (accessed 10 December 2013).

National Youth Agency (2013) *You're welcome*. Online. Available: www.nya.org.uk/you-re-welcome (accessed 11 December 2013).

NCB (2013) *Video shows young people 'talking health'*. Online. Available: www.ncb.org.uk/ news/video-shows-young-people-talking-health (accessed 11 December 2013).

NHS Employers (2010) *Appraisals and KSF made simple: a practical guide*, London: NHS Employers.

NHS Estates (2004) *HBN 23: hospital accommodation for children and young people*, London: The Stationery Office.

North Port Talbot (2008) *Participation strategy for children, young people & their families*. Online. Available: www.npt.gov.uk/PDF/candypp_participation_A4.pdf (accessed 10 December 2013).

Office of the Children's Commissioner (2011) *Tell the commissioner*. Online. Available: www. childrenscommissioner.gov.uk/issue_rooms/commissioner (accessed 10 December 2013).

Oxford Dictionaries (2013) *Definition of 'participation' in English*. Online. Available: www. oxforddictionaries.com/definition/english/participation?q=participation (accessed 10 December 2013).

Participation Works (2013a) *Early years*. Online. Available: www.participationworks.org. uk/topics/early-years (accessed 10 December 2013).

Participation Works (2013b) *What do we mean by participation?* Online. Available: www.par-ticipationworks.org.uk/resources/what-do-we-mean-by-participation (accessed 10 December 2013).

Prout, A. (2005) *The future of childhood: towards the interdisciplinary study of children*, Oxon: RoutledgeFalmer.

Royal College of Nursing (2013) *Lost in transition: moving young people between child and adult health services*, London: Royal College of Nursing.

Royal College of Paediatrics and Child Health (2012) *Involving children and young people in health services*, London: Royal College of Paediatrics and Child Health.

Schön, D.A. (1987) *Educating the reflective practitioner: toward a new design for teaching and learning in the professions*, San Fransisco, CA: Jossey-Bass Inc.

Treseder, P. (1997) *Empowering children and young people: training manual – promoting involvement in decision making*, London: Children's Rights Office and Save the Children.

UCLH (2011) *New children and young patients website for UCLH*. Online. Available: www.
uclh.org/News/Pages/NewchildrenandyoungpatientswebsiteforUCLH.aspx   (accessed
11 December 2013).

UCLH (2013) *Welcome to our hospital*. Online. Available: www.childrenandyoungpatients.
uclh.nhs.uk (accessed 11 December 2013).

Unicef (2013) *Fact sheet: the right to participation*. Online. Available: www.unicef.org/crc/
files/Right-to-Participation.pdf (accessed 30 July 2013).

Unicef United Kingdom (2013) *Children's rights*. Online. Available: www.unicef.org.uk/
Education/Rights-Respecting-Schools-Award/Childrens-rights (accessed 10 December
2013).

White, S., Fook, J. and Gardener, F. (2006) *Critical reflection in health and social care*, Maiden-
head: Open University Press.

Young Children's Voices Network (2009) *Listening as a way of Life*, London: National Children's Bureau.

11

LEADING THE PROMOTION OF PLAY AND RECREATION

Alison Tonkin and Irene O'Donnell

This chapter outlines how play and recreation can be promoted through the use of effective leadership skills. It raises awareness of the need for all people who work within health and care to undertake leadership roles, irrespective of their level or the job role that they perform. The process of leading small-scale projects is explored, together with case studies that show how this has been done in practice. The Healthcare Leadership Framework is discussed and its use as a tool for enhancing service delivery is promoted. Finally, guidance on how to access and use basic statistical information is also presented, which allows some of the needs of the local community to be identified and responded to.

Chapter objectives

By the end of this chapter you should have an awareness of:

- why the promotion of play and recreation as part of service delivery for children and young people is important;
- promotional projects that have been used to promote the role of play and recreation across differing disciplines;
- how the Healthcare Leadership Model can be used for promoting play and recreation;
- how to access and use basic statistical data as evidence for enhancing targeted service delivery at the local level.

THE NHS KNOWLEDGE AND SKILLS FRAMEWORK

Personal and people development

- Develop own skills and knowledge and provide information to others to help their development
  - Identifies development needs for own emerging work demands and future career aspiration
  - Offers help and guidance to others to support their development or to help them complete their work requirements effectively

Service improvement

- Appraise, interpret and apply suggestions, recommendations and directives to improve services
  - Identifies and evaluates potential improvements to the service
  - Presents a positive role model in times of service improvement
  - Enables and encourages others to suggest change, challenge tradition and share good practice with other areas of the trust

(NHS Employers 2010)

THE COMMON CORE OF SKILLS AND KNOWLEDGE

Multi-agency and integrated working

- Understand the value and expertise you bring to a team and that which is brought by your colleagues

Information sharing

- Make good use of available information, appraising its content and assessing what else might be needed
- Identify gaps in information

(CWDC 2010)

Introduction

In 2013 the National Association of Health Play Specialists (NAHPS) commemorated the fiftieth anniversary of the first employed hospital play staff in Brook Hospital, London (NAHPS 2013). Since then, the profession has grown and there are now over 1,000 registered play specialists across the United Kingdom, working together with, among others, play workers, youth workers and nursery nurses as part of play service teams. At a time when the role of play and recreation within hospitals and healthcare settings is strongly advocated, the play specialist profession sees itself under threat and is in danger of being marginalized as the competition for finite resources within the NHS increases. Play services within healthcare settings are being scrutinized in terms of whether the services they offer provide 'value for money'. This is not a new issue, as noted by Webster (2000), who posed the following question:

> The development and implementation of a professional play programme must be funded out of overstretched health budgets. But is play for sick children a luxury, to be offered as and when money allows, or is it an integral part of how we meet the specific needs of children in hospital and [the] community?
>
> *(Webster 2000: 24)*

So the challenge within this chapter is to try to identify why play services are under such threat and provide suggestions as to how play and recreation can be promoted at a time of fundamental change within the NHS itself.

Exploring the problem

Promoting the value of play and recreation for the holistic care of children and young people should be relatively easy. The value of play and recreation for children and young people within hospitals is well documented, with a rich history of advocacy through numerous government reports. However, there is also a history of such reports having limited impacts on subsequent practice due to slow or absent implementation.

Promoting the provision of play within hospitals was first noted in the 'Welfare of children in hospital' report by the Ministry of Health in 1959 (better known as the Platt Report). The Platt Report identified that the emotional care of children while in hospital needed to be considered and that facilities for play should be provided while children were in hospital. Although the Ministry of Health agreed with the 55 recommendations from the report, implementation was slow and it wasn't until 1961 that nursery nurses were identified as a possible group that could be responsible for play provision (Jolley n.d.). In 1971 the Department of Health and Social Security (DHSS) reiterated recommendations that had been made within the Platt Report, including the need to provide play and education for children while they were in hospital. In 1976 an expert group within the DHSS published a report specifically relating to the provision of play for children in hospitals, identifying the need for specially trained play staff and the provision of a dedicated play area (Jolley n.d.). In 1991 the Department of Health published the 'Welfare of children and young people in hospital', which noted that play and education services 'should' be provided and that all services should meet the holistic needs of the child or young person (Jolley n.d.).

The publication of the *National service framework for children: standard for hospital services* (Department of Health 2003) once again advocated the role of play and recreation, under the banner of child-centred services (Department of Health 2003). The routine provision of play and recreation opportunities to meet the basic needs of children was clearly promoted, for patients and their siblings. Daily access to a play specialist was recommended for children while they were in hospital, as well as encouraging the use of play techniques across the multidisciplinary team (MDT), with play specialists being asked to model techniques to other members of the MDT so they, too, could use play-related activities and resources within their practice as the child progressed through their personal healthcare journey (Department of Health 2003).

It is not only government reports that identify and promote the need for play and recreation within healthcare settings. In 1965 the National Association for the Welfare of Children in Hospital (NAWCH) was established, evolving from Mother Care for Children in Hospital, which was set up in 1961, with the aim of persuading hospitals that the recommendations from the Platt Report could work (Action for Sick Children 2013). In 1984 the NAWCH devised 'The Charter for Children in Hospital', which was designed to raise the quality of services provided for children within hospitals (Veerman 1992). The charter contained ten principles, the tenth of which stated 'Children shall have full opportunity for play, recreation and education suited to their age and condition' (Jolley n.d.).

This was the first charter of its kind and was approved by the Royal College of Nursing and the British Paediatric Association, but the principles were not legally binding and, therefore, there was no obligation to implement them (Veerman 1992). However, many of the same principles are now reflected within the European Association for Children in Hospital (EACH) Charter. For example, compare the principle above from the NAWCH Charter with principle 7 from the EACH Charter:

> Children shall have full opportunity for play, recreation and education suited to their age and condition and shall be in an environment designed, furnished, staffed and equipped to meet their needs.
>
> *(European Association for Children in Hospital 2013)*

EACH link many of their principles to articles from the United Nations Convention on the Rights of the Child (UNCRC), and these articles are legally binding following ratification of the Convention in 1991 by the UK government. Principle 7 of the EACH Charter specifically relates to Article 31 of the UNCRC, which states that 'every child has the right to relax, play and join in a wide range of cultural and artistic activities' (Unicef 2013). This means the delivery of play and recreational opportunities through the provision of appropriate facilities must be offered to children and young people while they are in healthcare settings, just as they should be in other areas of their lives.

So, five decades on from the Platt Report, is this the case in the modern NHS?

Activity 11.1

Most healthcare settings that deal with children and young people should be aware of the need to provide opportunities enabling play and relaxation, as stated in Article 31. The article also states that opportunities to join in a 'wide range of cultural and artistic activities' should also be provided.

Explore how your setting provides opportunities for artistic activities for:

- young children
- children aged 8–11 years of age
- young people.

Now consider how your setting provides cultural activities for the same age categories.

Knowing that this is technically a legal requirement under the UNCRC, if you have found that artistic and/or cultural activities are not being provided as part of the service provision for children and young people within your setting, why do you think this might be?

Sir Ian Kennedy was asked to undertake an independent review of the services being offered to children and young people by the NHS in 2010. Within specialist services for children and young people, Kennedy (2010) identified that the delivery of care by dedicated staff in dedicated facilities provided good experiences that were appropriate to the needs of the sick child being cared for. The role of play and distraction techniques was noted and the provision of youth workers was recognized by young people as an important aspect of their care. However, smaller centres or areas that lacked specialist facilities for children also lacked the specialist services that were seen as instrumental in providing positive experiences for children accessing health services. Kennedy noted that this was not necessarily the result of a lack of awareness of the value of play, but a matter of funding, stating that:

> The management of pain is often poor and I was told of at least two hospitals where play therapy services, so important as regards the experience children have of treatment, have recently been withdrawn for financial reasons.
>
> *(Kennedy 2010: 31)*

Therefore, it would appear the emotional value of play for children and young people's holistic development is now recognized and acknowledged, but the financial value of play in terms of service delivery is not. Kennedy (2010) goes on to suggest that additional services that provide high-quality, focused care for children and young people are the very services that are at constant risk from cost cutting measures as they do not in themselves show how they have contributed to the clinical outcome.

The NHS Leadership Academy has developed a new leadership model for the NHS (which is discussed later in the chapter). Initial research undertaken as part of this process proposed three main categories, one of which was the need to 'provide and justify a clear sense of purpose and contribution'. This focuses on the needs and experiences of people using the service and will require evidence of effective healthcare (Storey and Holti 2013). This need for evidence has also been identified in the *NHS outcomes framework 2013/14* (Department of Health 2012).

Chapter 9 explored how evidence of play service effectiveness and efficiency could be generated through the use of investigative techniques such as auditing or service evaluation. But more in terms of how play contributes to effective clinical outcomes will be required, especially as the commissioning of services becomes an established part of play service engagement.

Promoting the role of play and recreation

Clinical staff that utilize the services of the play team as part of their own clinical practice will often provide glowing testimonies about the benefits of integrated play techniques for the child, their family and the outcome of the intervention or procedure itself. Play input is now seen as an integral part of a care plan for children and young people who will be undergoing a course of radiotherapy (Royal College of Radiologists *et al.* 2012). This demonstrates how clinical recognition can be embedded into service delivery to maximize clinical outcomes and overall experience for the child or young person. Likewise, the benefits of play techniques for preparing children for anaesthesia are also well documented. For example, Armstrong and Aitken (2000) note that children who have been prepared for anaesthesia are calmer and more responsive than those children who have not been prepared. This suggests that clinical staff who have had a positive experience of play service involvement are usually advocates for play and will readily promote this service within their clinical practice. Recently, the president of the Royal College of Paediatrics and Child Health (RCPCH), Dr Hilary Cass, became patron of the NAHPS, which provides a major opportunity for promoting play to over 15,000 members of the College (Royal College of Paediatrics and Child Health 2013).

The examples above cover just a fraction of the children and young people's workforce within the health and care sector. The challenge is to raise the profile of play and recreation to a much wider audience.

Play in Hospital Week

Play in Hospital Week traditionally occurred every four years but recently, with sponsorship from the Starlight Children's Foundation, it has become an annual autumn event. Play in Hospital Week promotes the importance of play and provides an opportunity for play teams to 'showcase' their services. As 2013 was officially the fiftieth anniversary of employed play teams in hospitals, settings were encouraged to search their local archives to produce displays that showed how play has evolved since 1959. As part of this promotional activity, the NAHPS provided an activity pack that could be downloaded from their website (NAHPS 2013). As well as containing a range of age- and stage-appropriate activities that could be used with children and young people, it also contained printable posters that could be displayed covering topics such as:

- what health play specialists are;
- why play in hospital/healthcare is important;
- distraction therapy techniques.

These displays need to be seen by as many people as possible, so entrance halls, main corridors and canteen areas could all be utilized to maximize exposure. Presenting art and craft work undertaken by the children and young people themselves provides a ready source of colourful and unique display items, with the added benefit of enhancing children's self-esteem as their work is displayed. Children and young people were also encouraged to enter a creative competition linked to the theme '50 years of play in hospital', which also provided another source of artwork to be displayed.

There was also an information sheet entitled 'Getting play in the press' with tips, suggestions and offers of support from the Starlight Children's Foundation (2013) to enable this to happen. For many play specialists, the thought of engaging with the press can be daunting, so a template was provided to help play specialists make initial contact with the local press. There was also a series of featured articles and pictures within the professional journal for play specialists run by the NAHPS.

Informal methods of promoting play and recreation have also been used and Case Study 11.1 highlights how the NAHPS used Twitter to promote, publicize and share updates and information about what was happening across the country. Twitter is a microblogging service that comes under the banner of online social networking. It allows registered users to send and read text messages, called 'tweets', of up to 140 characters in length.

Other professional groups also promote their profession and this can be a good opportunity to work collaboratively to promote play and recreation as part of the celebration.

World Radiography Day

On 8 November 1895, Wilhelm Roentgen discovered X-radiation and this day is commemorated annually as World Radiography Day. Although this event is primarily designed to raise awareness of diagnostic imaging and radiation therapy, the Society and College of Radiographers provide promotional materials as a pack including stickers, posters and badges, which can be used as a starting point. Once again, requests were made for reports and images showing how departments celebrated the day, to be used in future editions of the professional magazine *Synergy News* (Society and College of Radiographers 2013).

Case Study 11.1

We know that social media is a widely used tool and a significant majority of the population engage in some form of social online activity on a daily basis. In recent years many well-known organizations have started to use social media to communicate messages to the public. For example, the Department of Health, the Royal College of Nursing and NHS England.

The NAHPS as a professional body have been reviewing ways in which we can further connect with both our members and other key organizations and decided to embrace the opportunities that social media can bring. The NAHPS Committee decided to register as Twitter users, enabling them to post and receive 'tweets'.

The first tweet was posted on 3 October 2013 and tweeted 'NAHPS is very excited to have joined twitter and would like to kick off with the countdown to Play in Hospital week' (NAHPS Committee 2013a).

Having started posting tweets, we soon realized what a fantastic tool this was to enable us to promote our profession and the value of play and recreation for people working in healthcare. We quickly followed all the key organizations that are relevant to children and young people's health. Re-tweeting by another Twitter user also increases visibility. With support from NHS England, they helped to re-tweet our posts and increase the number of followers, which helped share information about Play in Hospital Week. This included targeting specific organizations and settings that had Twitter accounts, asking them directly what their plans were for celebrating Play in Hospital Week. Significantly, this resulted in responses from many hospital trusts around the United Kingdom, who got in touch to tell us what they were doing, sending photos and stories about events and activities that were happening within their settings. This included settings that had previously not responded to any other means of communication. We have been able to share these tweets on our Twitter account, which makes promotion of events and activities much easier and also allows us to celebrate success.

> Thank you to all the #playspecialists who have sent NAHPS photos and stories on your celebrations for play in hospital week!
>
> *(NAHPS Committee 2013b)*

Targeting individuals who can share and endorse tweets is another advantage of using Twitter as a communication tool. For example, Dr Hilary Cass, president of the RCPCH and patron of the NAHPS, tweeted on the first day of National Play in Hospital Week: 'hugely important that we protect our play specialist workforce' (Cass 2013). While the NAHPS has 133 followers of their Twitter account, the RCPCH currently have over 3,200 followers who will have been able to access this tweet. If each of these Twitter users then re-tweet to their followers, it becomes clear that the opportunity to share is enormous.

Teddy Bear Hospital

Teddy Bear Hospital (TBH) is a medical school health project that runs across the country in conjunction with the European Medical Students Association.

> The project is aimed at young children between the ages of 5–7 years to help alleviate their concerns and anxieties about hospitals and doctors through fun activities and play.
>
> *(Teddy Bear Hospital – Leeds 2013)*

Medical students from the University of Leeds visit local schools, Beaver Colonies and Brownie Packs, and deliver workshops with a variety of stations that the children can visit. These include 'healthy eating, X-rays, basic First Aid, basic anatomy and introduction to the surgical theatre'.

Activity 11.2

Teddy Bear Hospital – Leeds have provided an overview of the format they follow when undertaking a school visit.

Access this at https://sites.google.com/site/teddybearhospitalleeds/what-we-believe

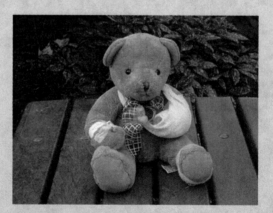

FIGURE 11.1 Pawly Bear having been 'treated' in a healthcare setting.

You can also watch some of the activities featured on YouTube – for example, the X-ray Station is shown at www.youtube.com/watch?v=2-aapW9PGo4

Although this is designed as a project for young children, what benefits do the medical students get from volunteering to be part of this programme?

How do you think this experience will impact on the medical students' clinical practice when they qualify?

One of the most noticeable features of all these promotional activities is the need for people to plan, organize and deliver these activities, usually in addition to their existing job role or student studies. Although ideas and resources can be accessed to help with the delivery of such projects, these projects need people to 'lead' the process.

The role of leadership within practice

Virtually any activity or event that requires decisions to be made by a group of people incorporates an element of leadership whereby someone 'takes the lead', usually in pursuit of a common goal.

The diverse nature of leadership and the scope of activities covered means the concept of leadership is difficult to define (Hendry 2013). Scouller and Chapman (2012) state leadership can be found in 'every sort of work and play, and in every sort of adventure and project, regardless of scale, and regardless of financial or official authority'.

Reflection

Think back to a time when you have watched a group of children playing together while engaging in imaginary play. Did you observe any dominant behaviour or a child 'taking the lead' within the children's play?

- What variables do you think determine which children exhibit dominant or leadership behaviour?
- How can this behaviour be supported and nurtured within your practice?

According to Bohlin (2000), young children demonstrate leadership and dominance strategies when playing with their peers. Predictor variables can be identified relating to age, gender, temperament and language development for individual children, while the length of time spent with peers, in terms of months, also determines the strategies children use when playing with their peers. Older children were able to demonstrate organizational leadership when interacting with peers and girls used prosocial behaviour (actions that benefit others) on more occasions than boys of the same age (Bohlin 2000).

The identification of leadership and dominance behavioural strategies by young children suggests there may be certain characteristics or traits that define leadership potential. Trait-based leadership was the dominant theory from the mid nineteenth century onwards, whereby leaders were 'born into the role'. However, a definitive and reliable list of distinctive leadership traits has not been forthcoming and it has been suggested that 'traits alone do not adequately explain what effective leadership is, nor how it can be developed' (Scouller and Chapman 2012). An alternative set of leadership theories focus on leadership styles and their associated behavioural skills and attitudes. This opens up the possibility of developing leadership potential through practice and training and broadens the pool of talent that is available.

Using the Healthcare Leadership Model to promote play and recreation

As an organization, the NHS promotes leadership as a shared responsibility and everyone can contribute to this process, albeit at differing levels. The NHS Leadership Academy (2011) asserts that all staff within NHS-funded health and care settings should aspire to be leaders, irrespective of their job role or level of employment. In 2013 the NHS Leadership Academy (2013: 3) developed the Healthcare Leadership Model to 'help those who work in health and care to become better leaders'. This applies to anyone who works within health and care, whether or not they have direct contact with 'patients and service users'. This new approach to leadership focuses heavily on 'leadership behaviours' and asserts that 'you will realise what you do and how you behave will affect the experiences of patients and service users of your organisation, the quality of care provided, and the reputation of the organisation itself (NHS Leadership Academy 2013: 3).

The Healthcare Leadership Model identifies leadership behaviours across nine 'leadership dimensions'. The context in which leadership is demonstrated is also an important factor and there is a four-stage scale which becomes more complex and sophisticated as leadership capacity evolves. The four stages are 'essential; proficient; strong; exemplary' (NHS Leadership Academy 2013).

Activity 11.3

A copy of *The Healthcare Leadership Model: the nine dimensions of leadership behaviour* can be accessed at www.leadershipacademy.nhs.uk/wp-content/uploads/2013/10/NHSLeadership-LeadershipModel-10-Print.pdf.

Explore the differing dimensions, reviewing and reflecting on how each area could be used to promote play and recreational activities.

Case Study 11.2 demonstrates how this has been applied in practice while promoting the role of play and recreation. It provides evidence that demonstrates effective leadership behaviour across a number of the nine dimensions and at different stages within each dimension. In particular, it links to the 'Engaging the team' dimension, which is important as leaders need to 'promote teamwork and a feeling of pride by valuing individuals' contributions and ideas; this creates an atmosphere of staff engagement where desirable behaviour, such as mutual respect, compassionate care and attention to detail, are reinforced by all team members' (NHS Leadership Academy 2013: 10).

It shows 'exemplary' leadership behaviour that addresses the following question: 'Do I create a common purpose to unite my team and enable them to work seamlessly together to deliver?' (NHS Leadership Academy 2013: 10).

Case Study 11.2

At present in the NHS we are all experiencing intensive changes, both economically and socially, due to the current climate. As managers we have increasing pressure to ensure the services we are providing are efficient and cost-effective, while being actively encouraged to source cost-saving measures and justify staff ratios and grades, and on occasion their very existence.

As the play services manager, I was asked to carry out a workforce review that needed to justify the staff banding and ratios within the play team. At the time there was no formal coordination of annual leave or study leave and teams tended to work in isolation within their own ward or department. To avoid job cuts or de-banding of posts it was imperative to show a change which was going to improve upon the current service provided without any additional cost implications.

A change to the current working patterns would allow the outcomes of being able to provide cross-cover of the service to avoid absence of service, coordination of leave to ensure staff levels were appropriate and the provision of an equitable service in all areas. Bringing about a change in this instance would enhance and improve the service, which is a fundamental factor in delivering change. It was noted that this change could not happen overnight and an appropriate time frame was set over several months, to include a consultation period, a trial period and review. The following action plan demonstrates how the change within the team's working patterns was planned and managed.

I used Lewin's 'Change Management Model' to structure the process. Lewin's model is based on the concept of unfreezing the current behaviour, introducing the change and refreezing when the change is accepted and becomes the new norm (Mindtools 2013). This process is outlined in Table 11.1.

For this change to be embraced and adopted it was necessary for me to work jointly with the team and as the leader of the change allowing them to fulfil their new roles, as opposed to managing them to do it. It was also imperative to lead by example and participate in the covering arrangements, which I did.

I used reflection as a model to help the team to analyse the current way of working and then after the trial period, the new way of working. In addition, one idea we used was staff shadowing each other before they had to formally cover an area to gain confidence and guidance from each other. One of the breakthrough moments for me was when a member of the team, who had been very resistant to the change initially, told me of her reflection on her positive experience of covering an area she had not worked in for some time and how much she had enjoyed it and gained from it – priceless!

TABLE 11.1 Action plan for managing change to team working practices

Detailed specific actions in sequence	Responsible person(s)	Resources	Date/time	Changes to look for
Step 1 Present the idea of change of working patterns – cross-covering and coordination of leave to the team, comparing it against the current way of working (Unfreezing stage)	Line manager	PowerPoint presentation setting out rationale for the change, staff meeting, information on current working negative impact	Early January 2012 12:30–13:30	Positive reactions, acknowledgement of need for change
Step 2 Consultation period with staff – opportunity to give feedback and comments on the change and time to digest the information (Unfreezing stage)	Line manager, all play specialist team, ward and department managers using the play service	Meetings, time to discuss, one to ones, introduce the idea at the senior managers meeting	Two-week period in January 2012	Positive reactions, acknowledgement and support of the need for change, reduction in anxiety and fear of change, gain acceptance
Step 3 Introduce staff rota for all leave and covering arrangements (Change stage)	All staff including line manager, senior play specialists	Office time to formulate a rota, dates of annual leave from staff, meeting time to discuss and plan, bleeps for staff to use as a contact	February 2012	Enthusiasm for change, resolve uncertainty and look for new ways
Step 4 Starting the cross covering (Change stage)	All staff including line manager	Bleep to be accessible for covering other areas	March 2012	Adopt the new behaviour, embrace new working pattern, recognize benefits
Step 5 Review the new working arrangements trial period (Refreeze stage)	All team including line manager, ward and department managers	Staff meeting	May 2012	Positive feedback, adoption of new working pattern, application of the change and outcomes being achieved
Step 6 Review the change of working and plan staff development day (Refreeze stage)	Line manager, all staff, senior play specialists who have volunteered to help organize the day	Venue, facilitator	Ongoing – date for review October 2012	Positive feedback regarding change, evaluate improvements, self-esteem and confidence increased reinforcing new pattern of working

Within the 'Evaluating information' dimension, demonstration of 'strong' leadership behaviour addresses the following question:

> Do I conduct thorough analyses of data over time and compare outcomes and trends to relevant benchmarks?
>
> *(NHS Leadership Framework 2013: 7)*

One of the most effective sources of data is statistical information and today these are readily accessible and usually free of charge (Community Voluntary Action Tameside 2013).

The role of statistics

Valid and reliable statistics are a powerful addition to any report or presentation. They can enhance the evidence when demonstrating service effectiveness and/or efficiency and they can identify local needs, thereby providing a focus for the targeting of resources or funding bids (Community Voluntary Action Tameside 2013). For example, in 2013 in comparison to the rest of England, the London Borough of Brent had a higher level of childhood obesity at 4–5 years and 10–11 years of age, a trend that has emerged since 2011. This was not the case in 2010, when relatively speaking, both age ranges were well below the national average (Child and Maternal Health Intelligence Network 2013). These statistics provide a persuasive argument for the targeting of resources within this local area, perhaps through the use of a TBH-style 'healthy eating' station, which could be offered by the play team as a commissionable service.

All this information can be readily accessed for any local authority from the Child and Maternal Health Intelligence Network, which sits within Public Health England. Child Health Profiles for the past three years can be accessed; these simply presented, four-page summaries provide a snapshot using key health indicators.

Activity 11.4

Find the Child Health Profile for your local authority using the following process.

Put Child Health Profiles in a general search engine such as Google or go to www.chimat.org.uk/profiles

Click on the 'Child Health Profiles – PDF reports' and a new window opens with an A–Z search facility. Click on the first letter from the name of your local authority and it will take you to all the local authorities beginning with that letter. Find the name of your local authority and click on your chosen data set.

Have a look at the data and think how you could use this information within your practice.

How could you use this data, bearing in mind the link to the 'Evaluating Information' dimension, from the Healthcare Leadership Model, to demonstrate leadership?

An interactive online version that allows you to compare the key indicators in other areas can also be used, but this is more complicated and may require practice to use effectively. There is also an iPhone and iPad app that can be downloaded for accessing child health profiles while 'on the move' (Child and Maternal Health Intelligence Network 2013). Similar profiles have been developed in Wales; these were introduced for the first time in the autumn of 2013.

Public Health England also provides annual regional health profiles at both local authority and county levels. This also has an interactive map facility for comparing indicators and creating maps and charts for local areas.

Another rich source of local data can be accessed through the Office for National Statistics (2013) 'Neighbourhood Statistics' webpages following the release of the 2011 census data sets. As long as you know your postcode, you can access a whole range of information ranging from 'crime and safety' to 'economic deprivation', 'housing' or 'health and care'. Once again, you can simply put the search term 'ONS neighbourhood statistics' into a general search engine and then select the link.

For information on specific topics such as obesity, physical activity and diet in England, or accident and emergency attendances in England, the 'NHS Information Centre for Health and Social Care' also provides open access to a range of statistical data. This sits within the data.gov.uk website, which was set up by the government to make data from all government departments available through a single, searchable database (data.gov.uk 2013).

Useful sources of information

Community Voluntary Action Tameside (CVAT): the Learning Zone provides some excellent factsheets under the 'Useful resources' tab, particularly the 'Evidencing success' factsheets at www.cvat.org.uk/evidencing-success

Using and handling data is an introductory course from the Open University. Section 3 provides a gentle overview of how to interpret and analyse data through the use of graphs: www.open.edu/openlearn/body-mind/health/public-health/using-numbers-and-handling-data/content-section-3.1

Child and Maternal Health Intelligence Network: www.chimat.org.uk

Regional Health Profiles for England at local authority and county levels: www.apho.org.uk/resource/view.aspx?RID=116449

Office for National Statistics neighbourhood statistics: www.neighbourhood.statistics.gov.uk/dissemination.

NHS Information Centre for Health and Social Care: http://data.gov.uk/publisher/nhs-information-centre-for-health-and-social-care

The Health and Social Care Information Centre, set up as a result of the *Health and Social Act 2012* in April 2013, is another source of reputable information and data for health and social care: www.hscic.gov.uk/searchcatalogue

Chapter 24, Play as a therapeutic tool, of *The Great Ormond Street Hospital Manual of Children's Nursing Practices*, edited by Susan Macqueen, Elizabeth Bruce, Faith Gibson. Published in 2012, this chapter provides an excellent overview of how play can be used as a therapeutic tool within the context of nursing practice.

NHS Leadership Academy, *How the Healthcare Leadership Model has been developed*. This provides an overview of how the new model was developed and the research that was undertaken before its launch: www.leadershipacademy.nhs.uk/discover/leadership-model/model-development.

References

Action for Sick Children (2013) *Our history*. Online. Available: http://actionforsickchildren.org.uk/our-history (accessed 2 December 2013).

Armstrong, T. and Aitken, H. (2000) The developing role of play preparation in paediatric anaesthesia. *Pediatric Anaesthesia*, 10(1): 1–4.

Bohlin, L. (2000) *Determinants of young children's leadership and dominance strategies during play*, thesis, Indiana University.

Cass, H. (2013) *Hugely important that we protect our play specialist workforce* (Twitter), 14 October. Online. Available: http://twitter.com/RCPCH_President/status/389711 492872142848 (accessed 24 November 2013).

Child and Maternal Health Intelligence Network (2013) *Child health profiles*. Online. Available: www.chimat.org.uk/profiles (accessed 2 December 2013).

Community Voluntary Action Tameside (2013) *Local statistics and where to find them*, Ashton-under-Lyne: Community Voluntary Action Tameside.

CWDC (Children's Workforce Development Council) (2010) *The common core of skills and knowledge*, Leeds: Children's Workforce Development Council.

data.gov.uk (2013) *Home*. Online. Available: http://data.gov.uk (accessed 2 December 2013).

Department of Health (2003) *Getting the right start: national service framework for children – standard for hospital services*, London: Department of Health.

Department of Health (2012) *NHS Outcomes Framework 2013/14*, London: Department of Health.

European Association for Children in Hospital (2013) *The 10 articles of the EACH Charter*. Online. Available: www.each-for-sick-children.org/each-charter/the-10-articles-of-the-each-charter.html (accessed 2 December 2013).

Hendry, J. (2013) Are radiography lecturers, leaders? *Radiography*, 19(3): 251–258.

Jolley, J. (n.d.) *The progress towards family centred care as expressed in some key reports here summarised 1959 to 1999*. Online. Available: www.hull.ac.uk/php/hesmjj/intro/pdfs/history/Reports.pdf (accessed 2 December 2013).

Kennedy, I. (2010) *Getting it right for children and young people: overcoming cultural barriers in the NHS so as to meet their needs*, London: Department of Health.

Mind Tools (2013) *Lewin's Change Management Model: understanding the three stages of change*. Online. Available: www.mindtools.com/pages/article/newPPM_94.htm (accessed 2 December 2013).

NAHPS (National Association of Health Play Specialists) (2013) *NAHPS National Play in Hospital Week: 14–20 October 2013*. Online. Available: http://nahps.org.uk/index.php?page=events (accessed 2 December 2013).

NAHPS Committee (2013a) *NAHPS is very excited to have joined twitter and would like to kick off with the countdown to Play in Hospital week* (Twitter), 3 October. Online. Available: http://twitter.com/nahpsofficial/status/385689938693324800 (accessed 24 November 2013).

NAHPS Committee (2013b) *Thank you to all the #playspecialists who have sent NAHPS photos and stories on your celebrations for play in hospital week!* (Twitter), 24 October. Online.

Available: http://twitter.com/nahpsofficial/status/393372885215358976 (accessed 24 November 2013).

NHS Employers (2010) *Appraisals and KSF made simple: a practical guide*, London: NHS Employers.

NHS Leadership Academy (2011) *Leadership framework*, Coventry: NHS Institute for Innovation and Improvement.

NHS Leadership Academy (2013) *Healthcare Leadership Model: the nine dimensions of leadership behaviour*, Leeds: NHS Leadership Academy.

Office for National Statistics (2013) *Neighbourhood statistics*. Online. Available: www.neighbourhood.statistics.gov.uk/dissemination (accessed 2 December 2013).

Royal College of Paediatrics and Child Health (RCPCH) (2013) *The college*. Online. Available: www.rcpch.ac.uk/what-we-do/college/college (accessed 2 December 2013).

Royal College of Radiologists, Society and College of Radiographers, Children's Cancer and Leukaemia Group (2012) *Good practice guide for paediatric radiotherapy*, London: The Royal College of Radiologists.

Scouller, J. and Chapman, A. (2012) *Leadership theories*. Online. Available: www.businessballs.com/leadership-theories.htm (accessed 2 December 2013).

Society and College of Radiographers (2013) *Claim your World Radiography Day pack now!* Online. Available: www.sor.org/news/claim-your-world-radiography-day-pack-now (accessed 6 October 2013).

Starlight Children's Foundation (2013) *NAHPS Play in Hospital Week 2013: celebrating 50 years of play in hospitals*. Online. Available: www.starlight.org.uk/wp-content/uploads/2013/08/PIHW-2013-pack_final.pdf (accessed 6 October 2013).

Storey, J. and Holti, R. (2013) *Towards a new model of leadership for the NHS*, NHS Leadership Academy.

Teddy Bear Hospital – Leeds (2013) *Welcome to Teddybear Hospital Leeds*. Online. Available: https://sites.google.com/site/teddybearhospitalleeds (accessed 2 December 2013).

Unicef (2013) *A summary of the United Nations Convention on the Rights of the Child*. Online. Available: www.unicef.org.uk/Documents/Publication-pdfs/UNCRC_summary.pdf (accessed 5 October 2013).

Veerman, P. (1992) *The rights of the child and the changing image of childhood*, Dordrecht: Kluwer Academic Publishers.

Webster, A. (2000) The facilitating role of the play specialist. *Paediatric Care*, 12(7): 24–27.

12

USING PLAY IN DIVERSE HEALTHCARE SETTINGS

Alison Tonkin with Joan Arton, Sonia Ciampolini, Christina Freeman, Sharon Aylott, Abi Warren, Marcia Gilkes, Rebecca Kirby and Carol Sullivan-Wallace

This final chapter draws together the main themes that have been explored and discussed within the previous chapters. It presents examples of how 'play' can be used in a range of different settings by a variety of healthcare practitioners. The chapter concludes with a look to the future and how the use of play and recreational activities and resources may be extended to enhance the provision of services beyond the children and young people's sector.

Chapter objectives

By the end of this chapter you should have an awareness of:

- how play can be used within differing healthcare settings;
- how the provision of play can be adapted to meet the professional objectives of the health- or care-related activity or medical procedure;
- the importance of sharing effective play-related practice across the multidisciplinary team;
- play as a fun activity that children naturally enjoy and will engage with, provided opportunities are appropriate and accessible.

THE NHS KNOWLEDGE AND SKILLS FRAMEWORK
Communication
- Adapts communication to take account of others' culture, background and preferred way of communicating
  - Accurate information given
  - Appropriate information given

Personal and people development
- Evaluates effectiveness of own learning/development opportunities and relates this to others
  - People feel responsible for developing their own expertise
    (NHS Employers 2010)

THE COMMON CORE OF SKILLS AND KNOWLEDGE

Child and young person development

- Draw upon personal experiences and other people's perspectives, to help you to reflect, challenge your thinking and to assess the impact of your actions
- Evaluate the situation, taking into consideration the individual, their situation and development issues

Multi-agency and integrated working

- You should actively seek and respect other people's knowledge and input to deliver the best outcomes for children and young people
- Have a general knowledge and understanding of the range of organisations and individuals working with children, young people, their families and their carers

(CWDC 2010)

Introduction

The Healthcare Leadership Model (NHS Leadership Academy 2013) identifies a range of leadership behaviours that reflect the values of the NHS and the evolving needs of the patients and communities it serves. One of the recurring themes appears to be the sharing of effective practice not just within teams, but across different disciplines and the organization as a whole. The following examples show how play has been used to enhance the effective provision of health and care from differing perspectives.

The first case study is a classic example that many practitioners will relate to and shows how the use of simple props and the right environment can be used to successfully engage the child.

Pure tone audiometry screening for five-year-old children in a clinical setting

Joan Arton, audiology nurse specialist

Pure tone audiometry is carried out following routine audiology screening sessions in primary schools. The initial screening result within the school setting may have been inconclusive or the child may have failed to identify one or more of the sounds. Following a referral by the school nurse who carried out the initial procedure, the child, accompanied by their parent or guardian, is offered an appointment in a clinic setting with an audiology nurse specialist. In the waiting room introductions are made, the child is identified and the relationship between the accompanying adult and the child established.

The layout of the room where the test is to take place is very important. The room should be light, clean and welcoming, with chairs arranged in a semi-circle.

Simple toys, together with drawing materials, are placed on a separate low table. A teddy bear is seated on a chair with earphones on, in a similar position to that which the child will be adopting. The room is set up specifically to ensure the child is made as relaxed and comfortable as possible with their surroundings. The teddy bear is an integral part of this procedure as it helps to reduce anxiety the child may have about putting earphones over their ears.

A short medical history is taken from the accompanying adult and the procedure is explained to the child in simple terms. Before the earphones are placed on the child a test tone is played to the child, familiarizing them with the sounds they are about to hear through the earphones. The tone is made using the audiometer and initially the child can see how the sounds are produced. However, during the testing the child is faced away from the audiometer so they are unaware of when the sounds are made, thus ensuring optimum accuracy. Earphones are gently placed on the child with the help of the teddy bear if necessary. Various tones are presented to the child using the audiometer, and the results recorded. When the sound is heard by the child, he or she pushes a button as a corresponding light appears on the audiometer. A firm matter-of-fact approach is taken during the audiology testing, followed by praise and a sticker at the end of the test.

If the child shows any distress the procedure is stopped and the parent/guardian offered another appointment. At no point should the procedure cause discomfort or fear. This may be the first time the child has had such testing in a clinical setting and the experience may affect subsequent visits, so it is important that the procedure should run smoothly and hold positive memories.

Another factor that may influence the approach taken by the audiology nurse specialist is the developmental stage of the five-year-old child. It may be appropriate for the child to sit on the lap of the accompanying adult. Most five-year-old children are able to press a hand-held button to signify that they have heard the presented tones. However, some may prefer to respond by placing small wooden bricks into an empty container. It is vital to engage the child in the testing procedure, to empower them and raise their self-esteem.

Results are discussed with the child and the parent/guardian with reference to a clear, printed diagram of the ear. An appropriate letter and an information booklet, together with a printed copy of the results, may be given to the parent/guardian and if necessary the procedure explained for a further appointment with an audiologist.

Activity 12.1

The pure tone audiometry screening process demonstrates a number of theories that have been applied in practice. Try to identify the different theories, noting how they may contribute to the screening process (most of these were covered in Chapters 4 and 5).

Hint: there are at least seven different theories from five different theorists.

The following account, written by a hospital interpreter, provides four examples that have indirectly influenced clinical activities through engaging children and young people with play opportunities.

Interpreting and play

Sonia Ciampolini, hospital interpreter (and registered health play specialist)
Working at a large teaching hospital, I have found opportunities to promote play for children within my work, without interfering with my job as an interpreter.

I interpreted for a lady at an antenatal clinic who brought her two-and-a-half-year-old daughter to the appointment. As we were waiting to be called by the obstetrician, the toddler became restless and kept trying to sit on her mother's lap, which was difficult as she was heavily pregnant. The girl looked bored, unhappy and frustrated. I offered paper and pencils, placing them on an empty seat next to us. At first she hesitated but soon started to scribble, changing coloured pencils and occasionally smiling at her mother. The doctor called us and the girl continued drawing in the room for a total of 25 minutes.

As I was interpreting for another lady who was consulting a gastroenterologist, her two-year-old son started tapping on her arm, interrupting the conversation, requesting things. Having got the doctor's permission, I asked the boy if he wanted to draw. He timidly agreed and I gave him paper and pencils. He scribbled using different colours, sharpened some pencils though this was not necessary, and played with the pencils. He calmly and happily entertained himself for over 20 minutes, calling his mother occasionally to blow her a kiss as she looked at him.

I interpreted for a lady coming for an ultrasound scan who brought her 27-month-old daughter. While mum stood by the bed having her legs scanned, the girl sat on a chair quietly holding her teddy bear. Soon she started fidgeting and touching the computer mouse. The sonographer looked at her disapprovingly. I then gave her a piece of paper and a pen (all I had). She stayed still, not a word. She gave me serious looks and I pretended not to notice. Gradually she grabbed the pen and released it, a few times. Then she grabbed the pen and scribbled lines at the bottom of the page. After a while, she left the chair and stood closer to mum and me. She started fiddling with the hospital equipment and I suggested making a bed for her teddy who 'looked sleepy'. I gave her a folded paper for a pillow and a bigger one for the blanket. She quietly took the things from me and went to the chair to 'arrange the bed'. By the end of the scan, she looked very sleepy herself when put in her pushchair to leave.

I interpreted for a 13-year-old boy with chronic constipation having sessions with a psychologist. He was very shy and introverted, and avoided socializing because of recurrent 'accidents'. As we waited in the children's outpatient waiting area, he was normally very quiet while mum vented her frustration at his condition with me, in front of him. On the third session, as they arrived ten minutes before the appointment, I decided to invite him to play table football with me, with the excuse that I wanted to play but felt embarrassed to play alone. He accepted and we played animatedly for about 15–20 minutes. I made the game competitive and he engaged well and laughed. I wanted to prevent him from listening to mum's negative remarks about him and to provide him with an opportunity to have normal play and fun. When the psychologist called us she looked at him and said she had never seen him looking so happy and in such a positive mood.

The next two examples show how collaborative working can benefit the health and care of children and young people through extension of traditional roles and areas of practice.

Radiography, play and recreation

Christina Freeman, professional officer; policy and guidance, the Society and College of Radiographers
Radiography is one of the Allied Health Professions, and radiographers are registered with the Health and Care Professions Council (HCPC). Radiographers are pivotal to delivering fast and reliable diagnoses of disease, and curative and palliative treatment and care for patients with cancer. There are two distinct categories of radiographers; diagnostic radiographers take the lead responsibility for the management and care of patients undergoing the spectrum of clinical imaging examinations, and therapeutic radiographers take the lead responsibility for the management and care of patients undergoing radiotherapy.

Radiographers work with patients of all ages from before birth (obstetric ultrasound) to after death (forensic post-mortem imaging). Engaging with babies, children and young adults forms a significant part of the workload for diagnostic radiographers and a small but significant part of the workload for therapeutic radiographers treating patients with cancer. On qualification all radiographers would have learned about child development and how to communicate with, and care for, children. However, this would only be a small part of the training programme and most newly qualified radiographers admit to feeling anxious about dealing with children. Radiographers working in specialist children centres undergo additional specific training, but most children are imaged in adult hospitals and radiographers are grateful for help and support given by healthcare colleagues, such as health play specialists, who are experts in the field of caring for children through the use of play.

At University College Hospital (UCH) in London, play specialists have been working with radiographers on a project to improve the imaging experience for children and their carers. Having a magnetic resonance imaging (MRI) scan is daunting even for adults; the machinery is large and noisy, but by having a dedicated play specialist the service for children has been transformed. The radiographer in charge of the MRI unit books children into a dedicated paediatric session and the play specialist is on hand to explain to the child and their carers exactly what is going to happen in an age-appropriate way. Colouring sheets, stickers and other resources help the play specialist prepare the child for the scan. The radiographers report that the child is more cooperative and the quality of the imaging is improved and hence the diagnosis is more accurate than it was before this project started.

Making the link between radiographers and play specialists has had other benefits at UCH and there are several joint projects underway. An area in the main imaging department is being transformed into a dedicated children's area and play specialists are involved, advising on the environment and what to include by way of child-friendly resources. Having play specialists available for the radiographers to talk to has led to greater understanding and the level of care and quality of the resultant images have improved significantly.

The Society and College of Radiographers (SCoR) is the professional body representing radiographers in the United Kingdom and it recognizes the value of its members working with play specialists as an expert group, as advocated within the *Practice standards for the imaging of children and young people* (Society and College of Radiographers 2009). The SCoR promotes good practice and encourages sharing. It uses its networks and website to encourage the radiography workforce to follow good practice as demonstrated at UCH.

The role of play in a specialist burns unit

Sharon Aylott, health play specialist

I work as a senior health play specialist on a specialist burns unit. Most of the children we see are under the age of two years, and within this group around 66 per cent are boys. Children's skin is far more sensitive and delicate than an adult's skin. A child can sustain a full thickness burn in just one second when exposed to water at 60 °C. The major cause of burns and scalds for children under five years of age is hot drinks; a cup of tea can still scald a child 15 minutes after it has been made.

I use play to normalize the hospital experience for the child, by promoting the use of play as part of the daily routine. I also use play to explain why the child is in hospital and what will happen while they stay with us. We do not use dolls or teddies due to infection control measures, but the child can bring their own in from home.

One of first things I do is explain to the child and their family what a dressing change is and I make this appropriate to each individual child depending on their age, developmental stage and their level of understanding. For children aged three years and under, I need to prepare the parents as much as the child as this can be a harrowing experience for parents, especially if there is associated guilt if they contributed to the child's injury. While preparing the child I use a special book that shows pictures of what they'll see and also use real bandages and equipment that will be used during the dressing change.

During the dressing change, I will offer distraction for the child. Pain and anxiety are linked and distraction has been shown to reduce anxiety, which in turn reduces the associated pain. I use resources that the child likes and that are fun. I also support the adult to support the child while their dressing is being changed. Sometimes distraction doesn't work and this means increased support for the parent is then also needed. It is beneficial for some children to hear a parent's voice rather than a member of staff.

Many children want to see the area that has been burnt and will watch what is happening. I help the child to cope and children generally cope well – but the parents may not. Parents will often try to divert the child's attention and when this happens, I help the parents to allow the child to watch. I will talk with all parents after their child's dressing change to see how they are feeling and if there was anything that maybe the parent and I could have done differently in supporting the child. Interestingly, parents that do not like their child seeing the burn wound have issues around how they are feeling in seeing the injury.

One of the problems with burns is the management of the scarring that will occur as a result. The occupational therapists and physiotherapists manage the physical aspects, but a scar will always be a constant reminder of the injury. Although the child may initially cope well once they have left hospital, when they reach puberty or a point of transition, for example moving from primary to secondary school, this may cause difficulties for the child as they look different to their friends and concerns about their body image arise.

Before the child and their parents leave the hospital, I prepare them for the future and provide some basic accident prevention and safety awareness work with the family. This usually means, depending on the age of the child, the use of safety gates and where to place hot drinks. We have extended this accident prevention work into an outreach project in the local community. We have seen a pattern about the lack of safety awareness and how to prevent burns. The main focus is raising awareness about food temperature and hazards around meal times. Hot drinks are the most likely cause of burns and scalds to children under the age of two and, aside from advising putting all hot drinks out of the reach of children, we give simple advice such as using safety mugs with sealable lids for hot drinks. We also promote the use of the Children's Burns Trust, which is a good source of information and advice. One of the most important pieces of information that we share with parents is the importance of first aid around the burn. Although often for the children that we see it can be too late, if this information can be passed on to other people such as parents, family members and staff working with children, it could make a remarkable difference in the outcome of treatment to a burn-injured child.

A big part of my role is also the management and coordination of the Burns Family Group.

This involves planning a variety of events throughout the year whereby children, siblings and their parents come together in sharing fun activities. These events may vary from a teddy bears' picnic in the park to a sleep-over at the Natural History Museum. These events may sometimes be age appropriate or for all the families to come together.

These events give the children opportunities to meet other burn survivors that have shared similar experiences. For parents it also gives them the opportunity to meet other parents that have experienced the emotional trauma of having a child with a burn injury. Lifelong friendships are often made during these events.

> ### Activity 12.2
>
> At a time when collaborative working is being promoted, the sharing of play-related practice is increasingly being transformed into commissionable services (as discussed within Chapter 9). Using the information above, how could the Healthcare Leadership Model be used to demonstrate leadership behaviours and what use may this be in promoting play-based services?

The next two case studies show the flexible nature of play provision and how its use can be planned and delivered within a range of community settings, including the child's or young person's home. The case studies come from Noah's Ark Children's Hospice.

Play in the Community: Noah's Ark Children's Hospice

Abi Warren, head of specialist care

Noah's Ark Children's Hospice provides hospice and family support services to life-limited and life-threatened children and their families living in north London, by helping families enjoy their lives together while their child is still alive or undergoing stressful treatment, and go on to face the future with hope if their child dies.

Our services have developed over time in response to the requirements of our families – we aim to provide what families say they want, when they want it and in a place of their choosing. Noah's Ark supports families by providing:

- a nurse-led team of specialist carers delivering sessions of care in the families' homes;
- a sibling support programme with bi-monthly fun activities focused around the needs of young people with a seriously ill brother or sister;
- specially trained family support volunteers who provide regular help for the families with all sorts of things from doing the shopping to helping with homework;
- a specialist play service working in the families' homes providing sessions which are fun and stimulating and help the children and their siblings cope with difficult feelings and worries;
- a family link team of experienced social workers to assess families' needs, help parents navigate complex service, care and benefits procedures and provide ongoing highly personalized one-to-one support at the end of the phone or in person;
- family days, parents groups and events to help tackle isolation, providing regular opportunities to get out and about and have fun with other families in similar situations.

Noah's Ark Children's Hospice believes that play is such a vital aspect of a child's life. We aim to ensure all of our staff and volunteers understand its value and importance by providing regular training, enabling us to integrate play into all the services and activities we provide.

Play Training for Home Support Volunteers

Marcia Gilkes, health play specialist, Noah's Ark Children's Hospice
As a play specialist in the community, I work within the families' homes to support children with life-limiting and life-threatening conditions, and their siblings. I support children who have anxieties or concerns around their treatment and children who have multiple sensory impairments. I also support their brothers and sisters in dealing with their siblings' condition and possible death.

One aspect of my role is promoting play within the organization, as well as providing training to our volunteers. As a charity, we rely on the help of volunteers to carry out many roles. Home support volunteers (HSVs) go into the child's home to befriend the life-limited or life-threatened child and/or their siblings, and provide practical and emotional support to the family where they need it most. In order to provide this support, the HSV must undergo intensive training, including a focus on play.

The main objective of the session is to teach the HSVs about the importance of play and to encourage and empower them to be equipped to play with children with varying needs within their own homes. The training covers five different areas.

My senses

While many children need support to play, children with sensory impairment, which can include a lack of movement, sight and hearing loss and sensitivities to touch and lights, often require extra support to access play. During the training the HSVs undergo an experiential session to gain an understanding of how it feels to have one or more senses removed. They are encouraged to use this experience when playing with children with sensory impairment and to take into consideration their tone of voice, where they position themselves in relation to the child, to talk to the child about what they are doing and what is going to happen and to always ask permission before giving or taking something from them, or offering a new activity.

What is play and why it is important

Looking at the value of play, and using the acronym SPICE (social, physical, intellectual, creative and emotional) I explain the importance of approaching play activities from a holistic perspective. I also explain how children with disabilities can experience play if we focus on their strongest abilities, as this can help them to develop new skills.

Stages of play

I try to give the HSVs an understanding of the typical developmental stages of play and explain that many of the children we work with may not have reached the expected milestones for their chronological age. We discuss the need to try to understand a child's developmental age and the importance of taking this into consideration when choosing play activities to use with them.

Sensory play and methods

The emphasis on 'sensory play' enables the children's learning and all-round development while allowing children with sensory impairments to have fun. Sensory impairment can affect the child's abilities, and in turn their self-esteem and self-confidence. There are many specialist toys that enable children with sensory impairment to access and enjoy play that most of the HSVs had not come across or experienced before. In order for them to feel confident in using these toys, and for them to be able to play effectively with the children, this session enables them to use the toys themselves and understand how they work. Using switch toys, LED lights and texture toys enables them to see the possibilities available to them and the children, and see how these specialist toys can help towards stimulating positive reactions and movements through touch, sound and vision.

Boundaries

Working within the child's home is very different to working in a public place, like a ward or a clinic. It involves us, as professionals, entering the child's space, and the child is able to be seen in their own environment, often with their entire family present, working around their normal day-to-day routine. It is vital that the HSVs understand their boundaries, and as part of their wider training they receive intensive training on this topic. However, it is also discussed in this session in relation to ensuring the HSVs are able to understand their responsibilities and limitations as to what they can deliver. They are also taught the need to explain to the child at the beginning of their session that, at the end, it will be put away. If HSVs have bought toys from Noah's Ark, they need to promote how to look after borrowed toys and what behaviour is expected. This helps the children to feel safe and form a trusting relationship with the HSV from the beginning.

The role of specialist carers and play

Rebecca Kirby, Noah's Ark Children's Hospice
As a specialist carer, I look after children from birth to 19 years old with life-limiting and life-threatening conditions. I bring fun, laughter and memories to families' lives. While providing respite for these children the main focus is play. I provide play for children in the child's home, at playgroups, on outings and at hospitals when they have appointments or are unwell. Play can happen at any time

while I am with a child, from a planned activity for their learning and development to during feeding, bath time and personal care, and it can also be used to distract the child during hospital procedures.

When preparing a session for a child it is important to know the child, understand what their condition is and what limitations this may cause. Some children are blind, so play is based around sound and touch, whereas other children are deaf so play is more visual. It is important to make the sessions fun so I incorporate what they like but it is also important to include things that help the child's development.

After taking these things into consideration and determining what we will do during the session I go into the office and select toys from the toy library. These might include sensory toys, adapted toys that can help a child communicate, things to smell, to touch, to listen to and to look at. I also get arts and crafts supplies for expression and even food for baking and messy play.

One of the children that I provide respite for has cerebral palsy. The child enjoys playing with their siblings, so I organize play activities that they can play together. Some of the games we have played include catch, football or balloon volleyball. We have had egg and spoon races, played twister or played with a bat and ball. These games are fun and encourage the children to work together. We also do a lot of arts and crafts such as papier mâché or hand painting, drawing or colouring in, which allow the children to be creative and express their feelings. When there are special occasions I have planned activities around these, such as pass-the-parcel and musical statues for a birthday, and pumpkin carving for Halloween. In the summer when the weather is nice we all go to the park and play there.

As well as playing with the siblings, when I am carrying out the care tasks that the child needs such as feeding, washing and dressing we will sing and play games. When the child is going to bed or is unwell the play will be a lot more calming to help the child relax and to make them feel better. This is when we may play with sensory lights or read stories and listen to music.

As a specialist carer I received training from a play specialist at the hospice and shadowed them to see how this works in practice. Additionally, I have been into the school the children attend, which gives me an invaluable insight into the way they play and learn.

Reflection

The provision of play opportunities that extends across the family is a feature of the HSV and the specialist carer roles. Do you ever watch how families interact within waiting areas, especially during a busy clinic or when appointments occur in school holidays?

Is there anything you could do to engage siblings before or during appointments?

Is this even something you should have to consider?

The final example shows how the provision of play experiences expands on the need for specialized training to use equipment in an appropriate and safe way. It also shows how this training can then be cascaded, provided there is ongoing support available for all concerned.

The role of play for promoting sensory experiences for children with complex needs

Carol Sullivan-Wallace, health play specialist

This case study will focus on Ruby (details changed to protect the child's identity), who came onto the main paediatric ward at five months of age and was there for several months. I chose Ruby for this case study both because of and in spite of her age. An older child with disabilities has obvious play needs; a younger child who does not have the constant input of the family is at risk of not bonding with their caregivers and this will also result in a lack of stimulation. On several occasions I heard Ruby described as a good baby who never cried unless unwell; alternatively Ruby could have been described as a child who, if allowed, could withdraw into herself.

Ruby was suffering from the side effects of a genetic disorder and had been in hospital since birth. Her symptoms included the narrowing of the trachea and cardiac problems. Ruby often became unwell suddenly and for the first eight months of life her family were unable to care for her within a family setting.

A series of play sessions and observations noted that Ruby was fully aware of the presence of others. Ruby appeared to have limited movement in her limbs and any movements tended to be spasmodic and linked to chest seizures. At six months Ruby was still immobile and failed to respond to the toys on offer, although she had begun to smile when being read to. Ruby also showed signs of anticipation, looking from the page of the book to the reader and waiting for the repetitive sounds that accompanied the stories.

The play team had recently acquired a sensory trolley and new observations of play sessions were made with special attention given to both positive and negative responses. Ruby was unable to visit our multi-sensory room, but by using the trolley we were able to make Ruby's room into a multi-sensory environment. Evidence suggests that staff untrained in the use of sensory equipment fail to deliver both fun and therapeutic play sessions and may even have a negative effect on the child or young person (Fowler 2008). With this in mind, training of both the play team and of some student nurses was arranged and delivered by senior staff from a local school that specialized in working with children with special needs. Multi-agency working is essential for continuation of care for children and young people with disabilities (Department for Education 2012). The cascading of skills means that training can now be delivered by the play staff to the wider team working with children and young people, with continued support from external teaching staff.

The play plan that was written for Ruby was adapted after two play sessions using observations that were made after each activity. A CD of world music was played in the background and each activity lasted for one music track. The tempo of the music was used to dictate the type of activity used. For Ruby the activities were:

- a projector
- a vibrating tube
- bubbles
- a space blanket
- mirrors
- textured balls

These activities were planned to flow and allow Ruby to anticipate what would happen next. The first activity was meant to stimulate and alert Ruby and the last activity was a relaxing one. Although the play plan was age/stage appropriate, we were mindful that children with special needs are often offered play for younger children (Lindon 2001). Any signs of inattention or boredom from Ruby and the activity would be altered to engage her attention again. By keeping to the plan Ruby became aware of the play order and was able to show anticipation. The play session would have been more inclusive if Ruby had been able to use interactive switches and hopefully she will be able to do this as she continues to develop. The space blanket was the first activity that Ruby reached her hands out to; this was an emotionally moving moment for the play specialist. The routine use of textured objects and vibration tube appeared to lead to a gradual desensitization of touch, especially on Ruby's legs which rarely had any other sensory input. It is worth noting that direct use of vibration appeared to be too stimulating for Ruby and the vibration tube was placed on either a bouncy chair or cushion under Ruby's legs to temper the effects.

Ruby's play plan was kept in her files to allow all staff to access it and when the sensory trolley was unavailable a box of sensory equipment was left in her room. Initially Ruby's family were unhappy with play equipment being left in the room. The play team used the family's concern as an opening to talk about the importance of sensory stimulation and normalizing play and Ruby's mother was included in at least one play session. Children with disabilities are often surrounded by the sights and sounds of a clinical nature. Ruby had already shown us how she responded to enthusiastic storytelling and was now laughing and smiling in anticipation of the animal noises that accompanied the story. Having her family join in with the play seemed to give them the confidence to play with their child, which they had previously not shown.

Activity 12.3

The role of observations and the significance of interdependence functions were discussed within Chapter 4, leading onto the development of play plans within Chapter 5. Identify the differing phases when observations and the recording of play plans occurred and what effect this had on the provision of play opportunities for Ruby.

The play team recently received a request from a general medical ward for the use of the sensory room for an elderly patient experiencing confusion. It was thought that the sensory environment could help calm this patient while stimulating other senses (Stepping Stones 2008). Although as a play team we agreed that this would be a useful form of therapy, the problems of infection control meant we were unable to accept this request. We did assemble a sensory box containing fibre optic lights and textured tactile objects to share with the ward and are waiting for feedback on the success of the equipment.

A view to the future

The extension of play service provision that has traditionally been focused on children and young people is an area that is worthy of further investigation. As seen above, play-based techniques are increasingly being used with older people. According to the Alzheimer's Society (2013) there are currently 800,000 people in the United Kingdom who have dementia and this figure is predicted to rise to one million by the year 2021. However, it is also noted from these statistics that currently only 44 per cent of people with dementia are actually diagnosed as having the condition.

Dolls have been used as a vehicle for therapeutic play for people with dementia. Although this is considered to be a relatively new method and its efficacy has not yet been established, it is suggested that doll therapy can lessen distress and offer comfort to people with dementia (Mitchell and O'Donnell 2013). However, there is some concern that this may not be appropriate, as some people consider the use of dolls to be degrading and it is suggested that more research is required before it should be used more widely (Mitchell and O'Donnell 2013). For people with mild to moderate dementia, a systematic review undertaken by Woods *et al.* (2012) has identified evidence that the use of 'cognitive stimulation' improves quality of life, with enhanced communication and interactions. Cognitive stimulation is designed to stimulate memory and thinking, through the use of adapted resources such as puzzles, event cards, word games and 'practical activities such as baking and indoor gardening' (Woods *et al.* 2012).

The other area that may be increasingly significant is the provision of services for people with autism. Although there is no register or exact count, it is estimated that around 700,000 people have autism, which equates to 1.1 per cent of the population of the United Kingdom (National Autistic Society 2013). The incidence is significantly higher in men by a ratio of 1.8 per cent as compared to 0.2 per cent for women, which reflects the childhood prevalence statistics (Wirral Joint Strategic Needs Assessment 2013). Although the degree of autism will vary significantly, there are two core features which are 'persistent difficulties with social communication and social interaction: and restricted, repetitive patterns of behaviour, interests or activities' (Wirral Joint Strategic Needs Assessment 2013: 1).

The challenges around social interaction and being able to engage with service provision may present a real threat to the individual. Once again, the extension of theoretical perspectives and adaptations to meet the needs of the individual can make a big difference. Dimensions (2013) now offers 'autism friendly screenings at over 250 venues in partnership with Cineworld, ODEON, Showcase and Vue cinemas' once a month for a selected film. The following concessions show how adaptations have been made that address some of the classic features of autism:

- 'The lights will be on low
- The volume will be turned down
- There will be no trailers at the beginning of the film
- You'll be able to take your own food and drinks
- You'll be able to move around the cinema if you like.'

(Dimensions 2013)

Perhaps this could be considered for clinical environments that heighten sensory experiences due to the bright lights, associated 'hospital smells' and high levels of noise, especially in reception areas and the main public areas. For people with autism all these features are present within standard waiting areas and may contribute to stress, anxiety and distress for both the patient and their caregivers, if they accompany the patient.

Majzun (2011) advocates the sharing of best practice from children's hospitals with adult facilities, stating that 'grown-ups need play too [as] it reduces stress by taking patients out of the mental space of being sick' (Majzun 2011: 211). He goes on to suggest that distraction may be even more important for adults than it is for children as adults may be aware of the severity of their illness and, therefore, the use of art, music and horticultural activities may help to address the emotional and cognitive needs of the patient. If this is the case, then play-based techniques such as preparation and distraction and consideration of environmental factors may also be transferrable to adult services.

Suggested answers to activities

Activity 12.1 (some suggested answers – you may have more)

- Reciprocal determinism – Bandura (layout of the room)
- Modelling behaviour – Bandura (teddy has earphones on)
- Simple explanation of test – Donaldson (manageable test the child can engage in)
- Experiential learning – Piaget (pre-operational stage and the use of concrete experiences – child can see the sounds being produced before the test is done)
- Small tasks within the overall task – Skinner (testing procedure broken down into smaller tasks)
- Positive reinforcement – Skinner (given praise and a sticker)
- Hierarchy of basic needs – Maslow (importance of self-esteem)

Activity 12.2

The obvious dimension to target is 'Evaluating information', whereby information has been used to inform the proposal for improvement. The 'essential' stage relates to the gathering of data and all four questions should be considered in terms of routine practice for all practitioners to demonstrate the efficacy of their service. This information then needs to be used to measure performance, which can then be used to spot future opportunities. Strong leadership behaviours have been identified within both examples, which show creative thinking. Being able to spot how play services can be used within seemingly unrelated areas of practice in both areas has led to collaborative ventures, in the case of the burns unit developing an outreach project to promote the prevention of the accidents which cause most of the admissions to the unit for children under five in the first place! Finally, this leads onto 'exemplary' leadership behaviour where improved pathways and systems have been developed (NHS Leadership Academy 2013). Other dimensions can also be used, in particular, 'Connecting our service', 'Engaging the team', 'Developing capability' and 'Influencing for results'.

Activity 12.3

- Observations were initially done as part of routine play sessions – identified toys being offered were not appropriate and reactions were seen when Ruby was being read to. Original play plan drawn up.
- Introduction of new sensory resources meant new observations using these resources was needed – for signs of positive and negative responses. Resulted in adaptation of play plan after two sessions to reflect observational data.
- Ongoing, informal observation during the play session and activities were adapted to ensure engagement – no alteration to the play plan and this was adhered to during the session. This enabled Ruby to anticipate as the routine remained the same.
- Inclusion of the family as part of the play plan following training from the play staff – this gave the family confidence and enabled them to play with Ruby.

Useful sources of further information

Alzheimer's Society: www.alzheimers.org.uk

Children's Burns Trust: www.cbtrust.org.uk/newsevents/index.shtml

MindStart: www.mind-start.com: this American website provides a range of activities that have been specifically designed for people with dementia and Alzheimer's. It also provides information and research findings relating to the role of cognitive stimulation and how the activities can be used to support this area of provision.

Noah's Ark Children's Hospice: www.noahsarkhospice.org.uk

The National Autistic Society: www.autism.org.uk

References

Alzheimer's Society (2013) *Statistics.* Online. Available: www.alzheimers.org.uk/statistics (accessed 8 December 2013).

CWDC (Children's Workforce Development Council) (2010) *The common core of skills and knowledge*, Leeds: Children's Workforce Development Council.

Department for Education (2012) *Multi-agency working.* Online. Available: www.education. gov.uk/childrenandyoungpeople/strategy/integratedworking/a0069013/multi-agency-working (accessed 7 December 2013).

Dimensions (2013) *Autism friendly screenings at ODEON.* Online. Available: www.dimensions-uk.org/support-services/autism-care/autism-friendly-screenings/autism-friendly-screenings (accessed 24 March 2014).

Fowler, S. (2008) *Multisensory rooms and environments: controlled sensory experiences for people with profound and multiple disabilities – a guide to controlled sensory experiences*, London: Jessica Kingsley Publishers.

Lindon, J. (2001) *Understanding Children's Play*, Cheltenham: Nelson Thornes Ltd.

Majzun, R. (2011) Coloring outside the lines: what pediatric hospitals can teach adult hospitals. *Pediatric Nursing*, 37(4): 210–211.

Mitchell, G. and O'Donnell, H. (2013) The therapeutic use of doll therapy in dementia. *British Journal of Nursing*, 22(6): 329–334.

National Autistic Society (2013) *How many people in the UK have autism?.* Online. Available: www.autism.org.uk/about-autism/myths-facts-and-statistics/statistics-how-many-people-have-autism-spectrum-disorders.aspx (accessed 8 December 2013).

NHS Employers (2010) *Appraisals and KSF made simple: a practical guide*, London: NHS Employers.

NHS Leadership Academy (2013) *Healthcare Leadership Model: the nine dimensions of leadership behaviour*, Leeds: NHS Leadership Academy.

Society and College of Radiographers (2009) *Practice Standards for the Imaging of Children and Young People.* Online. Available: www.sor.org/learning/document-library/practice-standards-imaging-children-and-young-people (accessed 6 December 2013).

Stepping Stones (2008) *Snoezelen® environments and individuals who are elderly and confused.* Online. Available: www.steppingstonesres.org/aging/013-snoe.htm (accessed 24 November 2013).

Wirral Joint Strategic Needs Assessment (2013) *Wirral JSNA Autism.* Online. Available: http://info.wirral.nhs.uk (accessed 9 December 2013).

Woods, B., Aguirre, E., Spector, A.E. and Orrell, M. (2012) Cognitive stimulation to improve cognitive functioning in people with dementia (Review). *The Cochrane Database of Systematic Reviews*, 2012: n.p.

INDEX

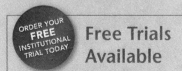
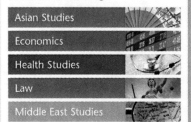